ULTRASOUND and AUTISM

What Every Pregnant Woman Should Know

ULTRASOUND and AUTISM

What Every Pregnant Woman Should Know

Jack Rabin, M.D.

Assisted by

Amy R. Kaufman

MEDICAL DISCOURSE
Autism Spectrum Disorder
2015

ISBN: 978-0-9825715-2-1

Library of Congress Control Number: 2014947826

Medical Discourse
PMB #451
5331 SW Macadam Ave., Suite 258
Porltand, Oregon 97239

PRINTED IN THE UNITED STATES OF AMERICA

Cover design by Paul Haist
Printed by Natural Press, Portland, Oregon

CONTENTS

ILLUSTRATIONS, CHARTS, AND GRAPHS

ABOUT THE AUTHOR

Jack Rabin, M.D., has practiced general medicine with an emphasis in neurology for 63 years in Long Beach, California. A multiply decorated veteran of World War II, he received his doctorate of medicine from the University of California–San Francisco Medical School in 1951. He received the Borden Prize in physiology for his research on the giant nerve fiber systems of the squid. In a contribution to the *Journal of the American Medical Association,* Dr. Rabin was among the first to alert the medical community that the original H_1N_1 vaccine, administered during the "swine flu" outbreak of 1976, was neurotoxic and caused paralysis later termed Guillain-Barré syndrome. In conjunction with his practice, Dr. Rabin conducted research on industrial neurotoxicology in his private laboratory. In retirement he is studying the etiology of the autism (ASD) epidemic.

In this book the term *fetus* is used to mean either *embryo* or *fetus*.
The fetal period starts with gestational week 11.
The term *operator* is used to mean sonographer, user,
end user, or clinician.

Introduction

This book was written to dispel the illusion of safety surrounding the use of ultrasound in pregnancy. An ultrasound examination, or sonogram, has become the first event in the medical history of virtually all unborn babies. Contrary to the advice of the American Institute for Ultrasound in Medicine, sonograms are performed repeatedly in low-risk pregnancies without a medical necessity. Most expectant parents are unaware that prenatal ultrasound is unsafe. The risks are not explained to them.

For 40 years, the use of prenatal ultrasound has increased exponentially, and each year the global autism epidemic has increased in parallel. The variations of autism, collectively known as autism spectrum disorder (ASD), result from a developmental abnormality of the fetal brain. Rapidly dividing brain cells are particularly susceptible to insult or injury by heating and other damaging effects of the ultrasound beam as it passes through fetal tissue. Scientific literature leaves no doubt that existing safety measures are inadequate to protect the fetus. Quoting from impeccable scientific sources, this book correctly describes the risks of prenatal ultrasound and presents evidence to prove that indiscriminate and excessive sonography is the cause of the epidemic of ASD.

The unremitting increase in the number of children with autism over the past 25 years is recognized as a global epidemic. According to a U.S. government report to Congress, the prevalence of autism in the United States increased by 500 percent from 1995 to 2005.[1] The U.S. Department of Education began to collect data on autism in the schools in 1991; the U.S. Centers for Disease Control (CDC) has published reports on the prevalence of ASD since 2000. The latest CDC report (2014) shows 1 in 68 U.S. children has been identified with ASD.[2] In some cases ASD is attributable to genetic factors, but genetic flaws by nature do not become epidemic. It is the belief of this author and other scientists that the progressive increase in ASD today is largely the result of a change in the environment of the unborn child. An external element is intruding on the protection of the womb, altering the development of the fetal brain.

The parallel rise of ASD and prenatal ultrasound has been discussed in the scientific literature for more than ten years. Prenatal ultrasound was introduced on a global scale in 1975, with the advent of ultrasound devices that could form clear images of the fetus during a sonogram.[3] Scientists have never ceased to warn that this powerful energy is hazardous to the fetal nervous system. In 1992 the U.S. Food and Drug Administration (FDA) permitted a nearly eightfold increase in the maximum intensity of ultrasound delivered to the fetus. For decades, ultrasound has been used more frequently, at higher intensities, and earlier in gestation, despite the warnings of international ultrasound safety organizations.

The existence of the autism epidemic refutes the claim that prenatal ultrasound has caused no observable harm. Drawing from the scientific literature, this book presents statistical and experimental evidence that proves today's epidemic of ASD is a result of prenatal ultrasound exposure.

- Autism has increased continually during the 23 years it has been tracked by governmental agencies. Autism was not recognized as a distinct disorder until 1943, when child psychiatrist Leo Kanner of Johns Hopkins University made the first precise study of the rare syndrome. Up to and including the Baby Boom (1946–1964), autism was believed to occur in fewer than 3 in 10,000 births.[4] Since the advent of commercially viable ultrasound machines in the mid-1970s, the prevalence of autism and associated neurological disorders (ASD) has steadily increased. According to the CDC, the prevalence of ASD increased from 1 in 150 U.S. children in 2000 to 1 in 68 in March 2014.[5] The preceding CDC study, conducted by a different method, reported a prevalence of 1 in 50 children.[6]

- The rise of ASD coincides with the increased use of prenatal ultrasound,[7] which is now universal in many countries. In virtually all of the four million U.S. births each year, the mother is scanned at least once and, on an average, four or five times.[8] Unlimited use has created a false assumption of safety. "In some countries, the number of prenatal ultrasound examinations has reached 10 per pregnancy,"[9] and there are no studies of the effect of cumulative doses of ultrasound on the fetus.

- Laboratory experiments have proved that prenatal ultrasound at current diagnostic levels "can produce temperature rises that are hazardous to sensitive organs and the embryo/fetus."[10] According to many scientists, existing precautions are inadequate to control exposure, and no assurance of safety can be made. The safety of the ultrasound exam is dependent on the operator, and studies have found most operators deficient in knowledge and training. Ultrasound physicists are working to resolve fundamental safety concerns that have persisted since the inception of obstetric ultrasound in 1957.[11]

Typically, an expectant mother is given a pamphlet with a reassuring statement such as the following: "To date, there is no evidence that diagnostic ultrasound produces harm in humans or the developing fetus when used properly."[12] The true meaning of this statement has been explained in the scientific literature. It means only this: Studies have found no *obvious* abnormalities that were evident to the naked eye at birth or shortly afterward; scientists have not yet *recognized* effects that can be *conclusively* attributed to ultrasound exposure. Physicians agree that microscopic, subtle, or delayed effects cannot be ruled out. There is no biological test or physical marker to detect autism in the womb or at birth[13]—only behavioral evidence that typically evolves and is observed in the developing child from two to twenty years of age. Autism spectrum disorder therefore corresponds to the medical definition of subtle or delayed effects.

No matter where they stand on the risks of prenatal ultrasound, physicians, scientists, and ultrasound safety organizations are united in opposing prenatal ultrasound for nonmedical purposes. In 2009 the European Federation of Societies for Ultrasound in Medicine and Biology (EFSUMB) issued the following statement:

> **Developments in real-time three-dimensional ultrasonic imaging have led to parents asking for souvenir (keepsake) video recordings of the fetus, sometimes at several stages during the pregnancy. . . . <u>[T]here are many instances of diagnostic scans being prolonged in order to provide such recordings.</u> . . . Very little information is currently available regarding possible subtle effects of diagnostic levels of ultrasound on the developing human embryo or foetus, and <u>the possibility of developmental effects in the brain cannot be ruled out.</u>[14] [Emphasis added]**

U.S. Food and Drug Administration

FDA Cautions Against Ultrasound "Keepsake" Images

by Carol Rados [excerpts from article in *FDA Consumer* magazine, Jan.-Feb. 2004]

[U]ltrasound is a form of energy, and even at low levels, laboratory studies have shown it can produce physical effects in tissue, such as jarring vibrations and a rise in temperature. Although there is no evidence that these physical effects can harm a fetus, **the FDA says the fact that these effects exist means that prenatal ultrasounds can't be considered completely innocuous.** [Emphasis added]

As more advanced ultrasound technologies (usually using higher ultrasound intensities) become available, greater numbers of expectant mothers and their families are requesting fetal keepsake videos and portraits for souvenirs. Sometimes these images may be made by people not well trained, or **for longer exposure times and at higher levels than are usually used in medical situations.** . . . [Emphasis added]

Besides concern that unskilled technicians could be performing and interpreting such ultrasounds and that the procedure is not always done under the supervision of a qualified physician, some facilities may be using equipment that's not in good working order. . . . [Emphasis added]

Exposure to ultrasound for longer than the time specified by the FDA for fetal monitoring could pose a **potential risk to the health of the mother and her developing fetus.**

[Full text of article is available at https://www.sdms.org/pdf/FDAKeepsake.pdf]

Physicians and scientists cite several reasons to avoid prenatal ultrasound in the absence of a valid medical indication:

- Ultrasound causes a rise in the temperature of fetal tissue directly attributable to "the transformation of one form of energy (sound) into another (heat)."[15] It has been established that "[d]eveloping tissues of the embryo and fetus are particularly susceptible to damage by heating, and the effects can have serious consequences."[16]

- Physicians and scientists concur that the practice of prenatal ultrasound should be governed by the principle of ALARA ("as low as reasonably achievable"). The mere existence of this guideline indicates an element of risk to the fetus. (See FDA warning, page 5.) ALARA is an inexact principle, best defined as follows:

  Until more adequate information is available, a prudent approach to using obstetrical ultrasound would be to obtain the necessary diagnostic information using the least possible exposure (a combination of intensity or power and time).[17]

- "It has long been thought that diagnostic ultrasound equipment could not produce biological damage. This assumption has *not* been supported by current research. . . . Our findings now suggest that the risk to humans is greater than previously thought."[18]

The Principle of ALARA
("As Low As Reasonably Achievable")

as defined by

the European Federation of Societies for Ultrasound in Medicine and Biology (EFSUMB)

EFSUMB Clinical Safety Statement for Diagnostic Ultrasound (2011)

The embryo/fetus in early pregnancy is known to be particularly sensitive. In view of this and the fact that there is very little information currently available regarding possible subtle biological effects of diagnostic levels of ultrasound on the developing human embryo or fetus, care should be taken to limit the exposure time and the thermal and mechanical indices to the minimum commensurate with an acceptable clinical assessment.

Quoted in *The Safe Use of Ultrasound in Medical Diagnosis* (2012), edited by Gail ter Haar, Ph.D., p. 150. This ebook is available at http://www.birjournals.org/site/book/Safe_Use_of_Ultrasound.pdf.

The leading ultrasound safety organizations have issued the following directives:

> (1) Prenatal ultrasound "scanning should be performed only with a valid medical indication."[19] "The use of ultrasound without a medical indication to view the fetus, obtain images of the fetus or determine the fetal gender is inappropriate and contrary to responsible medical practice."[20]
>
> (2) "[U]ltrasound should be employed only by health professionals who are trained and updated in ultrasound clinical usage and bioeffects."[21]
>
> (3) Ultrasound safety organizations and the FDA discourage the exposure of the fetus to ultrasound for the purpose of making "keepsake" or "souvenir" photos and videos. (See page 5.)

The safety of prenatal ultrasound is openly questioned in books that have recently been made available to the public. The 2012 edition of *The Safe Use of Ultrasound in Medical Diagnosis,* written by world experts in ultrasound physics and safety and "intended to be accessible to everyone," has been released as an ebook freely available for download. *Ultrasound: Medical Applications, Biological Effects, and Hazard Potential,* a 1987 work by international experts, was reissued in 2013.

Expectant mothers should be aware that the risk of prenatal exposure to ultrasound depends on many factors, including the stage of pregnancy, the intensity of the beam and how long it dwells on one part of the anatomy (dwell time), the vulnerability of the tissue on which the transducer is focused, the cumulative effect of exposure, the calibration of the equipment, and, to an exceptional degree, the expertise of the operator and the degree of his or her concern for safety. It is impossible to warrant safety in any of these respects. To date, there is no standard measurement of a dose of ultrasound.[22] We cannot accurately measure dwell time or the actual ultrasound-induced temperature increase in fetal tissue.[23] Few clinics check the manufacturers' calibration of ultrasound devices.[24] Jacques S. Abramowicz, M.D., member of the Bioeffects Committee of the American Institute for Ultrasound in Medicine (AIUM) and chair of the Bioeffects and Safety Committee of the World Federation for Ultrasound in Medicine and Biology (WFUMB), has described the "appalling" lack of knowledge of ultrasound operators.[25]

In the scientific literature it is often said that the use of prenatal ultrasound has outpaced research. Since the early 1990s, prenatal ultrasound has been used at higher and higher intensities without any evidence "to support the assertion of safety at these higher exposures."[26] As the studies quoted in this book will show, ultrasound is capable of inflicting brain injury that is later manifest in variations of ASD. The doctrine of ALARA is an attempt to abide by the first law of medicine: *Do no harm.* We have a duty to protect unborn children from unnecessary exposure to this form of nonionizing radiation, which, like x-ray, should be subject to stringent controls.

The text below appears in an advertisement for The Safe Use of Ultrasound in Medical Diagnosis, *published by the British Institute of Radiology. This 2012 book raises many of the safety issues concerning the use of diagnostic ultrasound in pregnancy. Retrieved from http://www.npl.co.uk/news/the-safe-use-of-ultrasound-in-medical-diagnosis*

The Safe Use of Ultrasound in Medical Diagnosis

The British Institute of Radiology (BIR), in conjunction with the National Physical Laboratory (NPL), the British Medical Ultrasound Society (BMUS), and the European Federation of Societies for Ultrasound in Medicine and Biology (EFSUMB), is making 'The Safe Use of Ultrasound in Medical Diagnosis' freely available for download.

The book, now in its third edition, is written for the practitioner and covers basic concepts important to the safe use of ultrasound and directs readers to extensive literature on the topic. It is edited by Dr. Gail ter Haar, who is currently chair of both the British and European committees for medical ultrasound safety, and team leader in the division of radiotherapy and imaging at the Institute of Cancer Research, London.

Adam Shaw, a Principal Research Scientist in NPL's Acoustics Group, is a member of the BMUS Safety Group and lead author of the chapter on 'The acoustic output of diagnostic ultrasound scanners'.

Sonographers and other practitioners increasingly need to be knowledgeable about the safety of a diagnostic ultrasound scan, as the onus has now shifted from the manufacturers to the person performing the scan.

President of the BIR, Professor Andrew Jones, said:

> "We hope practitioners in every hospital take advantage of
> this opportunity to update their skills online and without charge.
> As our new strategy gains pace we hope this first online
> eBook heralds a new vision in BIR publishing."

ENDNOTES

Introduction

1. United States Government Accountability Office (2005). Special Education: Children with Autism, Report to the Chairman and Ranking Minority Member, Subcommittee on Human Rights and Wellness, Committee on Government Reform, House of Representatives, p. 2. This report was a "Briefing for Staff of Rep. Dan Burton, Chairman, and Rep. Diane E. Watson, Ranking Minority Member, Subcommittee on Human Rights & Wellness, Committee on Government Reform, House of Representatives." Retrieved from http://www.gao.gov/new.items/d05220.pdf.

The graph on page 20 of this book shows the number of autistic individuals served by the U.S. Department of Education under the Individuals with Disabilities Act, "the primary federal law that addresses the unique needs of children with disabilities, including autism" (page 14, GAO report cited above). This book utilizes the same data source cited in the GAO briefing.

2. Centers for Disease Control and Prevention (2014). New data on autism spectrum disorder. Retrieved from http://www.cdc.gov/ncbddd/autism/data.html. It should be noted that the data published in 2014 are four years out of date and are undoubtedly underestimated.

3. Nicolson, M., and Fleming, J. E. (2013). *Imaging and Imagining the Fetus: The Development of Obstetric Ultrasound,* pp. 232-33. Baltimore: The Johns Hopkins University Press.

4. "The early autism surveys show a clear convergence in disease frequency from the 1950s through 1980, with four different studies reporting rates consistently lower than 3 per 10,000." Blaxill, M. F. (2004). What's going on? The question of time trends in autism. Public Health Reports, November-December 2004, vol. 119, p. 548.

5. The CDC's methodology for developmental disability surveillance was applied to ASD "following concerns about increases in autism during the mid-'90s," according to its report "Prevalence of the Autism Spectrum Disorders (ASDs) in Multiple Areas of the United States, 2000 and 2002," p. 15. The estimate of 1 in 150 is found on p. 18. Retrieved from http://www.cdc.gov/ncbddd/autism/documents/autismcommunityreport.pdf. The estimated prevalence of 1 in 68,

reported in March 2014, is based on eight-year-old children whose parents or guardians lived in 11 U.S. sites monitored by the CDC's Autism and Developmental Disabilities Monitoring Network in 2010. The U.S. Centers for Disease Control and Prevention (2014). New data on autism spectrum disorder. Retrieved from http://www.cdc.gov/ncbddd/autism/data.html.

6. The estimated prevalence of 1 in 50 is derived from the National Center for Health Statistics State and Local Area Integrated Telephone Survey 2011-2012 National Survey of Children's Health, p. 2. Retrieved from http://www.cdc.gov/nchs/slaits/nsch.htm. The survey is conducted by the CDC.

7. Abramowicz, J. S. (2012). Ultrasound and autism: Association, link, or coincidence? *Journal of Ultrasound in Medicine,* vol. 31, p. 1261.

8. O'Keeffe, D. F., and Abuhamad, A. (2013). Obstetric ultrasound utilization in the United States: Data from various health plans. *Seminars in Perinatology,* vol. 37, no. 5, Abstract. Retrieved from http://www.ncbi.nim.nih.gov/pubmed/24176148. doi:10.1053/j.semperi.2013.06.003

9. Abramowicz, J. S. (2010). Fetal Doppler: How to keep it safe. *Clinical Obstetrics and Gynecology,* vol. 53, no. 4, p. 845.

10. Ter Haar, G. (2012), citing the 2011 EFSUMB Clinical Safety Statement for Diagnostic Ultrasound, in *The Safe Use of Ultrasound in Medical Diagnosis,* p. 149. London: The British Institute of Radiology. Retrieved from http://www.birjournals.org/site/book/Safe_Use_of_Ultrasound.pdf.

11. Nicolson, M., and Fleming, J. E. (2013). *Imaging and Imagining the Fetus: The Development of Obstetric Ultrasound,* p. 225. Baltimore: The Johns Hopkins University Press. "Despite the failure of substantial research efforts to confirm any deleterious effect, the safety concern surrounding obstetric ultrasound was never quite laid to rest. Throughout the years covered by this book—and, indeed, until the time of writing—anxieties about possible hazards continued."

12. Nelson, T. R., Fowlkes, J. B., Abramowicz, J. S., Church, C. C. (2009). Ultrasound biosafety considerations for the practicing sonographer and sonologist. *Journal of Ultrasound in Medicine,* vol. 28, p. 139.

13. "ASD is currently diagnosed based solely upon behavior, with no validated biomarkers to aid in the diagnosis." The Interagency Autism Coordinating Committee (2012). Skafidas, E., Testa, R., Zantomio, D.,

Chana, G., Everale, I. P., and Pantelis, C. Predicting the diagnosis of autism spectrum disorder using gene pathway analysis, cited in *2012 IACC Summary of Advances in Autism Spectrum Disorder Research,* pp. 1-2. Retrieved from the U.S. Department of Health and Human Services Interagency Autism Coordinating Committee website: http://iacc.hhs.gov/summary-advances/2012/index.shtml.

14. European Federation of Societies for Ultrasound in Medicine and Biology (2009). European Committee of Medical Ultrasound Safety (ECMUS), Statement on the Use of Diagnosic Ultrasound for Producing Souvenir Images or Recordings in Pregnancy. Retrieved from http://www.efsumb.org/ecmus/souvenir-scanning-statement.pdf.

15. Abramowicz, J. S. (2002). Ultrasound in obstetrics and gynecology: Is this hot technology too hot? *Journal of Ultrasound in Medicine,* vol. 21, no. 12, p. 1327.

16. Church, C. C., and Barnett, S. B. (2012). Ultrasound-induced heating and its biological consequences, in *The Safe Use of Ultrasound in Medical Diagnosis,* p. 46. Retrieved from http://www.birjournals.org/site/book/Safe_Use_of_Ultrasound.pdf.

17. Fisher, B. R., and Stratmeyer, M. E. Developmental and teratogenic effects of ultrasound, in Repacholi, M. H., Grandol, F. M., and Rindi, A., eds., *Ultrasound: Medical Applications, Biological Effects, and Hazard Potential,* p. 213. New York and London: Plenum Press, 1986, reissued 2013.

18. O'Brien, W. D., Jr. (2001). Physical mechanisms for ultrasound-induced lung hemorrhage bioeffects, in *Medical Ultrasound Bioeffects,* second paper, p.1. Retrieved from http://www.icacommission.org/proceedings/ICA2001Rome/7_06.pdf.

19. Abramowicz, J. S. (2008). Bioeffects of obstetric ultrasound for the clinician: How to keep it safe, p. 1. Institute for Advanced Medical Education. Retrieved from https://iame.com/online/bioeffects_of_obstetric_ultrasound/content.php.

20. American Institute of Ultrasound in Medicine (2012). AIUM Official Statement: Prudent Use in Pregnancy. Retrieved from http://www.aium.org/ Click on Resources, click on Official Statements, select Safety. AIUM is a multidisciplinary society of over 7,500 physicians, sonographers, and scientists dedicated to the safe and effective use of ultrasound.

21. World Federation for Ultrasound in Medicine and Biology (2012). WFUMB/ISUOG Policy Statement on Souvenir Imaging of the Fetus. Retrieved from http://www.wfumb.org/about/statements.aspx.

22. Ter Haar, G. (2012). Chapter 1, *The Safe Use of Ultrasound in Medical Diagnosis,* p. 2. Ter Haar states: "A problem that has bedeviled the study of ultrasound bio-effects is the lack of a consistent method of describing 'dose.'"

23. Abramowicz, J. S. (2008). Bioeffects of obstetric ultrasound for the clinician: How to keep it safe. Institute for Advanced Medical Education. Retrieved from https://iame.com/online/bioeffects_of_obstetric_ultrasound/content.php. On p. 2 Abramowicz states: "One aspect that is absent from all calculations but that is vital if one wants to perform accurate and complete ultrasound dosimetry, is information on exposure time, including dwell time. . . . It is important . . . to note and remember that no epidemiological data available include dwell time. . . . nor do any of the existing exposure indices (thermal and mechanical indices) . . . take time into account." He continues on p. 6: "It needs to be made very clear that *TI* [the Themal Index] *does not represent an actual or an assumed temperature increase.* It bears some correlation with temperature rise in degrees Celsius such that a higher TI can be assumed to be associated with a higher temperature rise than a lower TI, but does not allow an estimate or a guess as to what that temperature change *actually* is in the tissue."

24. Francis A. Duck, Ph.D., D.Sc., writes: "The measurement of radiation is central to the tradition of radiology. The success of diagnostic ultrasound has resulted in the introduction into healthcare of very large numbers of ultrasound scanners. . . . Current hospital practice makes little or no attempt to evaluate the ultrasound radiation generated by this equipment. . . ." Duck, F. A., Ultrasound exposure measurement: A hidden science? *The British Journal of Radiology* (2005), vol. 78, p. 291.

25. Abramowicz, J. S. (2007). Editorial: Prenatal exposure to ultrasound waves: Is there a risk? *Ultrasound in Obstetrics and Gynecology,* vol. 29, p. 366.

26. Duck, F. A. (1999). Is it safe to use diagnostic ultrasound during the first trimester? *Ultrasound in Obstetrics and Gynecology,* vol. 13, p. 385.

U.S. DEPARTMENT OF EDUCATION STATISTICS

U.S. Children and Adults with Autism, Ages 6-21 Served under the Individuals with Disabilities Education Act, Part B (50 States, Washington, D.C., and Puerto Rico), by School Year (1991-2013)

School Year	Children with Autism
1991-1992	5,415
1992-1993	15,580
1993-1994	19,058
1994-1995	22,780
1995-1996	28,827
1996-1997	34,101
1997-1998	42,511
1998-1999	53,576
1999-2000	65,396
2000-2001	78,717
2001-2002	97,847
2002-2003	118,602
2003-2004	140,920
2004-2005	165,552
2005-2006	192,643
2006-2007	224,594
2007-2008	258,305
2008-2009	292,818
2009-2010	333,234
2010-2011	370,011
2011-2012	406,957
2012-2013	443,562

This table shows the increase in autism in the U.S. at a glance. The same data are represented on the graph on page 20, which includes sources and commentary.

I

The Parallel Rise of Autism and Obstetric Ultrasound

Scientists have long suspected that prenatal exposure to ultrasound is an environmental cause of autism spectrum disorder (ASD), a group of neurodevelopmental conditions that cannot be attributed entirely to genetic factors.[1] There has been an alarming increase in ASD since the late 1970s, with an attendant rise in the use of prenatal ultrasound, which has been widely used since 1975.[2] Autism is believed to originate in the human brain before birth; therefore, to find the source of the epidemic we must examine changes in the environment of the fetus over the past 30 years. Scientists have proved ultrasound energy is capable of damaging and disrupting the development of the fetal brain in mammals. It is unethical to perform experiments on human fetuses; therefore, we may never have conclusive, anatomical evidence that ultrasound is a direct cause of ASD. This is not a reason to disregard the compelling statistical evidence compiled by U.S. governmental agencies. This evidence establishes that the strong correlation between the increased use of ultrasound in pregnancy and the rise of ASD is more than a coincidence; it is a cause-and-effect relationship.

The parallel rise of autism and the use of prenatal ultrasound has been discussed in recent scientific literature. In his 2012 paper, "Ultrasound and Autism: Association, Link, or Coincidence?" Jacques S. Abramowicz, M.D., the obstetrician/gynecologist who chairs the World Federation for Ultrasound in Medicine and Biology (WFUMB) Bioeffects and Safety Committee, recognizes this parallel increase:

> **[I]t is clear that ASDs represent a major health problem in the world. . . . Although one can find a definite parallel increase in the prevalence of autism and the use**

antenatal ultrasound in the last 2 decades, an obvious question bears asking: . . . is there a causal relationship between these two phenomena; or is it pure coincidence?[3]

Autism is often described as a "once-rare disease."[4] Autistic symptoms were scarcely mentioned in medical literature until 1943, when American psychiatrist Leo Kanner, considered the father of child psychiatry, first portrayed the essential features of a condition he was to name *early infantile autism.* His 11 patients showed an "extreme aloneness from the very beginning of life, not responding to anything that came to them from the outside world," and "an anxiously obsessive desire for the maintenance of sameness that nobody but the child himself may disrupt."[5] Kanner's definition prevailed until 1980,[6] when autism was first listed as a separate entity in the *Diagnostic and Statistical Manual of Mental Disorders (DSM)* of the American Psychiatric Association. The diagnostic criteria have been revised several times since then. Today, in the fifth edition of *DSM (DSM-5,* 2013), Kanner's autism and similar conditions, such as Asperger's disorder, are encompassed by a single term: autism spectrum disorder (ASD). Manifestations of ASD "vary greatly depending on the severity of the autistic condition, developmental level, and chronological age; hence, the term *spectrum.*"[7]

Until 1980, autism was believed to occur in fewer than 3 in 10,000 children in the U.S.[8] ASD now affects at least 1 in 68 U.S. children, according to the March 2014 estimate of the U.S. Centers for Disease Control (CDC).[9] In testimony before Congress in May 2014, the United States Government Accountability Office (GAO) reported that from fiscal years 2008 through 2012, federal agencies spent a total of approximately $1.4 billion on autism research and related activities.[10] In 2012 Autism Speaks announced the estimated economic cost of ASD in the U.S. was $126 billion per year, "a number that has more than tripled since 2006."[11] According to a 2014 report, the annual cost of ASD in the U.S. is an estimated $175 billion.[12]

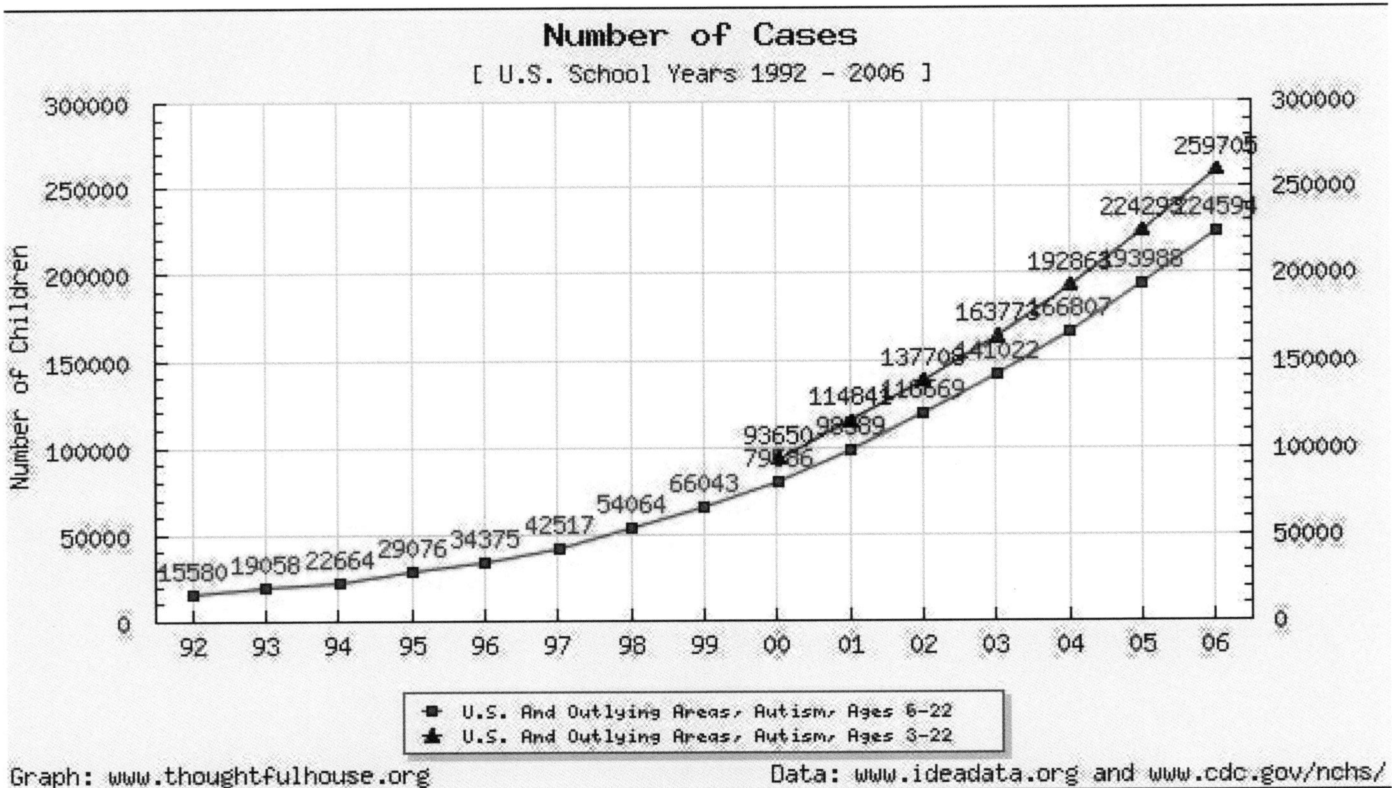

This chart, created by Thoughtful House, represents the number of autistic children age 6 to 22 (1992-2006) and 3 to 22 (2000-2006) who were served by the U.S. Department of Education under the Individuals with Disabilities Education Act. The data were derived from statistics published by the U.S. Department of Education and the U.S. Centers for Disease Control. The chart on the following page extends the Department of Education statistics to 2013 for children age 6 to 21.

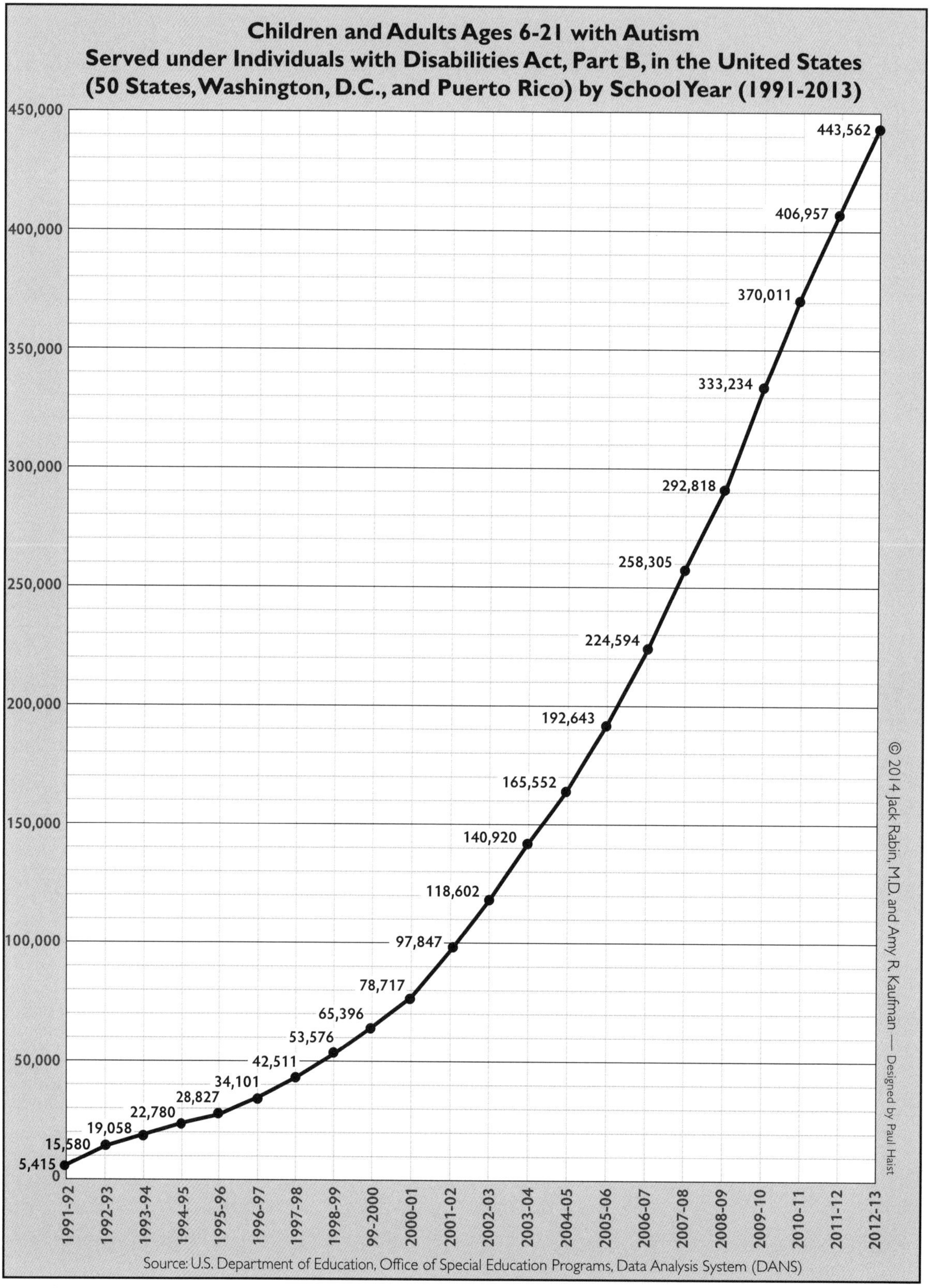
Children and Adults Ages 6-21 with Autism
Served under Individuals with Disabilities Act, Part B, in the United States
(50 States, Washington, D.C., and Puerto Rico) by School Year (1991-2013)
450,000
400,000
350,000
300,000
250,000
200,000
150,000
100,000
50,000
0
5,415
15,580
19,058
22,780
28,827
34,101
42,511
53,576
65,396
78,717
97,847
118,602
140,920
165,552
192,643
224,594
258,305
292,818
333,234
370,011
406,957
443,562
1991-92
1992-93
1993-94
1994-95
1995-96
1996-97
1997-98
1998-99
99-2000
2000-01
2001-02
2002-03
2003-04
2004-05
2005-06
2006-07
2007-08
2008-09
2009-10
2010-11
2011-12
2012-13
Source: U.S. Department of Education, Office of Special Education Programs, Data Analysis System (DANS)
© 2014 Jack Rabin, M.D. and Amy R. Kaufman — Designed by Paul Haist

The graph opposite provides a way to visualize the continual steep rise of ASD. The data are published in the U.S. Department of Education's Annual Report to Congress on implementation of the Individuals with Disabilities Education Act. It should be noted that the statistics in each annual report are approximately two years old by the time they are published; the figures are often revised after publication; and the figures reflect only those individuals enrolled in Part B of the Individuals with Disabilities Education Act (IDEA), not all individuals diagnosed with autism. Individuals with mild symptoms remain undiagnosed, and the most severely afflicted are unable to attend school.

Students with autism served under IDEA were first counted as a separate category in school year 1991-92. The graph includes school years 1991-92 to 2012-13, the last year for which statistics were available at the time of writing. There are differences between the charts on pages 19 and 20. The Thoughtful House chart on page 19 combines data from both the U.S. Department of Education and the U.S. Centers for Disease Control for children ages 6-22 and 3-22. The graph opposite represents data from the U.S. Department of Education only and includes children ages 6-21. The Department of Education's 2005 Annual Report to Congress explains the representation of age groups as follows: "Because the 1986 Amendments to EHA (now IDEA), P.L. 99-457, ended the practice of collecting data on children from birth through age 5 by disability, the information in this section refers only to children age 6 through 21."

Data through 2010-11 were obtained from U.S. Department of Education, Office of Special Education Programs, Data Analysis System (DANS), OMB #1820-0043: "Children with Disabilities Receiving Special Education Under Part B of the Individuals with Disabilities Act." These data are now difficult to access. Data for school years 1992-93 and 2001-12 were retrieved on 22 Aug. 2013 at http://www.ideadata.org, a site that no longer exists. Data for school years 1993-94 to 1998-99 were retrieved from http://www2.ed.gov/about/reports/annual/osep/index.html. Data for school year 2012-13 were originally retrieved in March 2014 by following the link to "2011-12/Fall 2012 IDEA" at http://www.ideadata.org/tools-and-products. Data for 2011-12 and 2012-13 could only be confirmed by personal communication with a representative of Westat, who sorted the data at https://inventory.data.gov.

The Exponential Increase in ASD

Statistics are "the first point to consider in any analysis of a disease or a condition."[13] As the charts and graphs in this chapter illustrate, the number of individuals with ASD in the U.S. has risen unabated since 1991. Experts agree that this phenomenon cannot be explained by genetic factors and must have one or more environmental causes.[14] Government agencies responsible for gathering data on ASD include the U.S. Department of Education and the U.S. Centers for Disease Control and Prevention (CDC).

The U.S. Department of Education provides special education programs for students with disabilities under the Individuals with Disabilities Education Act (IDEA). Each year the Education Department is required to submit a report to Congress on the implementation of this act. The "child count" tables include the number of students served, according to age and disability. Autism first appeared as a category of disability in school year 1991-92. From school years 1991-92 to 2012-13, the number of autistic individuals age 6-21 served under IDEA, Part B, increased from 5,415 to 443,562. (See pages 16, 19, and 20.) It should be noted that these data underestimate the number of children affected by ASD, documenting "only the children served, not all of the children who meet diagnostic criteria."[15] Appropriate education programs for children with ASD are not available in every state and school district. "For example, many children with autism have communication problems, but some school districts have encountered difficulties in providing speech and language services because of shortage of specialists who can provide these services."[16] As noted in *DSM-V*, ASD frequently co-occurs with one or more conditions, and diagnoses may overlap:

> **Abnormalities of attention (overly focused or easily distracted) are common in individuals with autism spectrum disorder, as is hyperactivity. . . . Many**

individuals with autism spectrum disorder have psychiatric symptoms that do not form part of the diagnostic criteria for the disorder (about 70% of individuals with autism spectrum disorder may have one comorbid mental disorder, and 40% may have two or more comorbid mental disorders).[17]

In 2000 the U.S. Centers for Disease Control and Prevention (CDC) designated several geographical sites in the U.S., called the Autism and Developmental Disabilities Monitoring Network (ADDM), for the study of ASD prevalence. M. Yeargin-Allsopp, M.D., a medical epidemiologist and chief of the developmental disabilities branch of the CDC, explains that the CDC estimates *prevalence* of ASD instead of *incidence* because "there is a great deal of variability in when a child actually manifests symptoms and then is diagnosed with an ASD":

The ADDM Network reports ASD prevalence, or the total number of children with an ASD at a specified age in a specified year per 1,000 children in the population. The ADDM Network does not use incidence because incidence is based on cases where a clear onset time can be documented. Typically, the onset of an ASD is not known, although it usually manifests by the time a child is 3 years of age.[18]

The CDC's 2012 report, reflecting the prevalence of ASD in 8-year-old children living in the 14 ADDM communities in 2008, was 1 in 88.[19] Later that year, the CDC announced the prevalence of ASD had reached 1 in 50, according to data gathered by the CDC's National Survey of Children's Health utilizing a different method:

Based on parent reports, the prevalence of diagnosed ASD in 2011-2012 was estimated to be 2.00% for

> **children aged 6-17. This prevalence estimate (1 in 50) is significantly higher than the estimate (1.16%, or 1 in 86) for children in that age group in 2007.[20]**
>
> **The reported prevalence of ASD has increased in recent decades. For example, data from the Centers for Disease Control and Prevention's (CDC) National Health Interview Survey (NHIS) revealed a nearly fourfold increase in parent-reported ASD between the 1997-1999 and 2006-2008 surveillance periods . . . . and CDC's Autsm and Developmental Disabilities Monitoring (ADDM) Network revealed a 78% increase in ASD prevalence between 2002 and 2008.[21]**

The CDC statistics underestimate the number of children with ASD. Its ADDM communities, numbering fewer than a dozen, represent only a small sampling of the population; the data are derived from interviews granted by parents or guardians of 8-year-olds only; and the CDC's annual reports are outdated by the time of publication. The 2014 estimate of 1 in 68 is four years out of date; however, the lag time between data collection and publication can be much longer. In their article "When 1 in 150 Is Really 1 in 67," Raymond W. Gallup and American pediatrician F. Edward Yazbak argued that the CDC's 2007 report grossly underestimated the prevalence of ASD:

> **Most people and the press have been under the impression that in the United States, the "new" CDC-reported prevalence rate of 150 was a recent discovery that was current for 2007 when indeed it was not at all. The study did not document a prevalence of 1 in 150 among children born now or five years ago. The study revealed that among U.S. children born in 1994,**

thirteen years ago, 1 in 150 on average had a spectral disorder.[22] **[Emphasis added]**

Assuming the 2007 statistics were correct, the authors contended, "it is likely that among children born in 2000 who are now registered in U.S. schools, the prevalence rate of autistic spectral disorders is around 1 in 67, on average. *Now that would be a catastrophe of unprecedented proportions.*"[23] [Emphasis added] It should be noted that this is almost exactly the prevalence we have reached today.

"The global prevalence of autism has increased twentyfold to thirtyfold since the earliest epidemiologic studies were conducted in the late 1960s and early 1970s," according to the 2014 CDC report on ASD prevalence.[24] This report specifically mentions the sharp increases in U.S. prevalence: The 2014 estimate (based on 2010 data) was 29% higher than the 2012 estimate (based on 2008 data), 64% higher than the estimate based on 2006 data, and 123% higher than the estimate based on 2002 data.[25] Increases of this magnitude would certainly rule out genetic changes as a cause of the autism epidemic. There is disagreement as to which year marks the beginning of the accelerated increase and what percentage of these cases is attributable to genetics, changes in diagnostic criteria, and environmental determinants, meaning any external factor that intrudes on the baby in the womb. However, most statistical studies concur that the prevalence of ASD is on an upward trend, and that genetics, changes in diagnostic criteria, and improved detection do not entirely account for the increase.[26]

ASD in America is now "recognized as the second most common developmental disability, after mental retardation, among children,"[27] according to the CDC. One physician wrote that autism had become "of great concern to the practicing pediatrician because of an astonishing 556% reported increase in pediatric prevalence between 1991 and 1997."[28] There was a "near exponential increase in the number of cases of autism in the U.S. between the years 1992 and 2007."[29] Dr. Yazbak, describing the rise of ASD as "the silent epidemic," spoke of its impact on the education system in 2008: "The arrival of nearly half the new enrollees to U.S. schools with 'high-severity disabilities,' many of which are related to the autistic spectrum, is a tidal wave unlike any other."[30]

Increased Usage of Ultrasound and Exposure at Higher Intensities

Ultrasound physicist William D. O'Brien Jr., Ph.D., states that although "[a]n important consideration with respect to the evaluation of risk is an estimate of the extent of ultrasonic exposure which the patient receives," risk is difficult to evaluate because "(1) the number of examinations a patient receives is generally unknown, (2) multiple examinations may be performed with different types of equipment, and (3) the amount of ultrasonic energy that a patient receives varies from exam type to exam type and from examiner to examiner."[31] The failure to accurately record each exposure also makes it difficult to assess the extent of use. However, there is evidence of a massive increase in use from 1971 to the present.

In his 1984 paper focusing on the safety of ultrasound in obstetrics, O'Brien reported that two surveys of selected U.S. hospital systems, conducted in 1971 and 1974 by the FDA's Bureau of Radiological Health, demonstrated "an almost 200% increase in use" between the surveys. The 1971 survey "found that 12% of the hospitals used diagnostic ultrasound.(10) The same Federal agency reported on the conduct of its 1974 hospital survey that 35% of the surveyed hospitals used diagnosic ultrasound.(11)" The 1974 survey "showed that an estimated 16% of the obstetric services in the United

States used diagnostic ultrasound and that about one-third of all U.S. births for 1974 were delivered in these hospitals. Additionally, it was estimated that 470,000 pregnant women were exposed to diagnostic ultrasound in that year with about 35-50% of these women being examined more than once."[32]

Summarizing the data on both increased sales of diagnostic ultrasound equipment and extent of use, O'Brien predicted in 1984:

> **[I]f one were to estimate that about one-half of all pregnant women are currently being examined with ultrasound and, additionally, that its usage is increasing at an annual rate of 10-25%, then within a few years, virtually every fetus could be examined with ultrasound.**[33]

O'Brien's prediction evidently was correct. Douglas L. Miller, Ph.D., wrote in 2008, "The exposure to diagnostic ultrasound in obstetrics occurs for virtually every mother and fetus in the developed and developing world."[34]

The number of ultrasounds per pregnancy is also increasing. A 2013 survey of data from various U.S. health insurance plans reported:

> **There is currently a lack of published data on ultrasound utilization in obstetrics in the United States. In order to get some meaningful information on this topic, we analyzed de-identified data obtained from large insurance providers and underwriters that covered [a] large segment of the United States population in various geographic areas of the country. Our results show an overall significant increase in utilization of obstetric ultrasound over the years, with pregnancies receiving around 4-5 ultrasounds per pregnancy.**[35]

Prenatal ultrasound is a medical diagnostic tool intended to facilitate the diagnosis of suspected major fetal anomalies. However, Miller observes, "The exposure of mother and fetus often occurs in routine examinations with minimal specific medical indication."[36] In the early 1990s the National Institutes of Health funded a major study to determine whether routine sonograms in low-risk pregnancies are beneficial to the child. This study of 37,505 women, known as the Routine Antenatal Diagnostic Imaging with Ultrasound (RADIUS) trial, found: "Routine scans do not seem to be associated with reductions in adverse outcomes for babies or in health service use by mothers and babies."[37]

How did the excessive, routine, unnecessary use of prenatal ultrasound take root in American obstetrics? Physicians Filly and Crane explain that by the time the NIH funded the RADIUS study, prenatal ultrasound had already become entrenched:

> **Importantly, many obstetricians in the United States had already made their own value judgment by this time and had instituted programs of screening in their practices. Indeed, it is fair to state that some practitioners had already concluded that if 1 sonogram during pregnancy was "good," then 2 sonograms were "better," and 3, 4, or 5 sonograms were "best." . . . Thus, by the time the NIH study results were published, the issue had already taken on a major financial impact in American obstetrics. Any result other than an overwhelming endorsement of routine sonography was certain to meet with a backlash.**[38]

Tariq A. Siddiqi, M.D., voices concern about repeated ultrasound exposure early in pregnancy:

> **[O]f the 4 million infants born in the United States annually, almost all are exposed to diagnostic ultrasound**

> **in utero. When assisted reproductive technologies are used, human embryos may be exposed to as many as 4 to 6 times in the first trimester. Such exposures carry the potential for bioeffects that may not appear for decades.**[39]

In the following statement Abramowicz estimates the alarming increase in power of advanced modes of ultrasound:

> **It is a reasonable assumption that most pregnancies in the U.S., and virtually all of them in many countries, are scanned with ultrasound. Most often, this is with regular gray-scale B-mode, but often color imaging and spectral Doppler modes are used, which have much higher acoustic energy outputs <u>(possibly by a factor of 100 or 1000).</u>**[40] **[Emphasis added]**

The popularity of "souvenir" or "keepsake" images and videos is one of the most glaring examples of excessive use of ultrasound. Following its 2010 Symposium on Safety of Nonmedical Use of Ultrasound, the World Federation for Ultrasound in Medicine and Biology (WFUMB) recommended: "In the absence of supporting evidence of safety, caution should be used to minimize ultrasound exposure to the fetus. . . . Because the safety of an ultrasound examination cannot be assured, the use of ultrasound without medical benefit should be avoided."[41] The International Society for Ultrasound in Obstetrics and Gynecology (ISUOG) specifically mentions the ignorance of nonmedical ultrasound operators and their tendency to focus the beam on the baby's face, which, this author contends, endangers the vulnerable fetal brain:

> **Major issues are the general lack of knowledge of end-users regarding the safety and bioeffects of ultrasound (21), the possible extended amount of time needed to**

obtain the "ideal" face image, as well as the unknown effect (if any) of cumulative exposure.[42]

The cause-and-effect relationship of prenatal ultrasound and ASD can be depicted in a few words:

In the 1950s obstetric ultrasound was in its infancy. From 1954 to the late 1950s, the cumulative incidence of autism in the U.S. was less than 3 in 10,000 children. Until the early 1970s, obstetric ultrasound was available in only a few medical centers.

With the advent of real-time scanning in 1975, ultrasound scanners became commercially viable, and they sold in an "exponentially" expanding global market for the next 20 years.[43] ASD was on the rise in the 1980s, and increased to more than "30 per 10,000 children in the 1990s, a 10-fold increase," according to Mark Blaxill's study.[44] The U.S. Environmental Protection Agency identified a spike, or "changepoint," in ASD prevalence in 1988-89,[45] known as the "autism boom."

In 1992 the FDA increased the allowable output of ultrasound devices used in obstetrics nearly eightfold, raising concerns for the safety of the fetus. From 1992 to 2007 there was a "near exponential increase in the number of cases of autism in the U.S."[46] From 1995 to 2006 the average number of prenatal ultrasound scans in the U.S. increased by 80 percent.[47] On the 50th anniversary of the American Institute for Ultrasound in Medicine in 2003, its president stated that by some estimates "more than 80 million ultrasound exams are performed annually in the United States."[48]

The following Chronology of Use of Ultrasound in Obstetrics provides a historical perspective on the development of ultrasound in obstetrics, which the reader may interpret in the context of the ASD epidemic.

Chronology of Use of Ultrasound in Obstetrics*

*The primary source of the information used to create this chronology is *Imaging and Imagining the Fetus: The Development of Obstetric Ultrasound,* by Malcolm Nicolson and John E. Fleming (Baltimore: The Johns Hopkins University Press, 2013).

1957 The first known ultrasound images of the human fetus are made in Glasgow, Scotland, in a team led by Ian Donald, M.D., a professor of midwifery at the University of Glasgow.

1958 Donald, the leading figure in the development of obstetric ultrasound, publishes a historically significant paper in *The Lancet* containing images of the fetus made with a bed-table contact scanner.

1959 First commercial sale of one unit of the new Automatic Scanner.

1963 Donald and his colleagues have "used the Automatic Scanner to examine more than 130 women whose pregnancies were of less than 20 weeks' duration."

1964 The Diasonograph scanner is first used at the Queen Mother's Hospital in Glasgow. By 1966, 12 Diasonographs have been sold to hospitals in England, North America, Iraq, and Scotland.

1965 Joseph Holmes, M.D., father of ultrasound in the U.S., hosts an international symposium on diagnostic ultrasound in Pittsburgh. In 1966 the first postgraduate course in diagnostic ultrasound is held at the University of Colorado Medical Center.

1972 The NE4102 ultrasound scanner is launched. "It was bought by many British hospitals, often as their first ultrasound machine, and was also sold widely throughout the world." During the next few years, "diagnostic ultrasound was being adopted by an increasing number of centers throughout the developed world."

1973	Advanced Diagnostic Research (ADR), an Arizona-based company, introduces the first "commercial real-time scanner that incorporated linear-array technology." Ultrasound machines become a highly marketable item.
1975	An improved model, the 2130, is launched. "Soon, every hospital in the developed world had to provide an ultra-ultrasound service. Indeed, before long, most obstetric clinics deployed several machines. . . . [A]s new models were successfully produced by Smiths Industries and Nuclear Enterprises, the scanners became more of a market commodity."
1975-1979	ADR sells 5,000 units of its 2301.
Late 1970s and 1980s	"The improvement in the quality of the ultrasonic image achieved in the late 1970s and 1980s allowed, for the first time, characterization of the soft tissue of the major fetal organs." Ultrasound machines are "standardized products in a high-volume global market." "Many maternity units began to offer routine scans at around 20 weeks, often in addition to an earlier booking scan."
1981	More than 4,000 new ultrasound machines are bought in the United States alone. "The market continued to expand exponentially throughout the next two decades."

The prevalence of ASD has risen in synchrony with the increased ues of ultrasound in pregnancy and the increased power of ultrasound imaging devices. When the fetal brain is subjected to the focused heat and other stresses of ultrasound, the trajectory of neurodevelopment can be altered. This eventually produces behavioral symptoms that vary according to the intensity of the beam, the parts of the brain exposed, the duration of exposure, the stage of gestation, and other factors. The autism described by Kanner is a disease of unchanging incidence. It constitutes only a part of today's ASD. The "autism spectrum" is pervading all societies where prenatal ultrasound is practiced. It may look like the autism of the past, but this is a new disease with a different cause.

Leading ultrasound scientists and obstetricians have repeatedly called for studies of the effects of prenatal ultrasound on the human fetus. Abramowicz laments the "paucity of rigorously conducted epidemiological studies to evaluate adverse outcomes of DUS [diagnostic ultrasound] in humans."[49] He proposes the ideal experiment: "Large epidemiological studies with half of the population exposed to ultrasound *in utero* and half not exposed would be the only way to demonstrate a clear effect or lack thereof."[50] In the U.S., such a comparative study would be infeasible because prenatal ultrasound is now virtually universal. Fortunately, two vast populations in the U.S.—one exposed to prenatal ultrasound, the other unexposed—exist in nature. The experiment advocated by Dr. Abramowicz has already been performed.

For centuries, unborn babies were not exposed to ultrasound. Autism was rare in the generations prior to and including the Baby Boom (1946-1964). Until 1980, when obstetric ultrasound devices had become a global commodity, autism occurred in fewer than 3 in 10,000 individuals. Autism is now a part of almost every family. More than 1 in 68 children in the U.S. have been diagnosed with ASD. The dramatic contrast between the unexposed and exposed populations has been ignored. The relative absence of ASD in the 78 million Baby Boomers compared to the vast increase of ASD in exposed fetuses is statistically observed evidence that medical exposure of the fetal brain to ultrasound is the cause of the soaring incidence of ASD. This is not a genetic disease; it is a manmade epidemic.

ENDNOTES

I. The Parallel Rise of Autism and Obstetric Ultrasound

1. Rosenblatt, A. I., and Carbone, P. S., Eds., with Yu, W. What causes autism disorders? in *Autism Spectrum Disorders: What Every Parent Needs to Know.* (Elk Grove Village: American Academy of Pediatrics, 2013), p. 25. The authors state: "In about 15% of children with an ASD, the condition is associated with a clear underlying cause such as a chromosome abnormality, a genetic syndrome, or a known environmental cause. In most children, however, the underlying cause of the ASD is not obvious."
2. Nicolson, M., and Fleming, J. E. E. (2013). *Imaging and Imagining the Fetus: The Development of Obstetric Ultrasound.* (Baltimore: The Johns Hopkins University Press, 2013), p. 232.
3. Abramowicz, J. S. (2012). Ultrasound and autism: Association, link, or coincidence? *Journal of Ultrasound in Medicine,* vol. 31, p. 1266. In this paper Abramowicz, one of the leading authors on the risks of prenatal ultrasound, addresses the possible connection between ultrasound and autism. An international expert in obstetric and gynecologic diagnostic ultrasound with special expertise in ultrasound bioeffects and safety, he is the author of 156 publications in peer-reviewed scientific journals.
4. Swedish psychiatrist Christopher Gillberg, a leader in autism research, wrote in 2005: "For a long time, childhood autism was considered to be an extremely rare disorder, with its prevalence rate usually reported at a fraction of a 10th of 1% (Lotter 1966; Brask 1970; Sponheim & Skjeldal 1998). . . . The most recent estimates of the prevalence of autism have ranged from 0.5% to 1.1%, that is, 20-100 times higher than those suggested in text books even in the mid 1990s (Lord & Rutter 1994)." Gillberg, C., The epidemiology of autism, in *The Neurology of Autism* (Oxford University Press, 2005), p. 119.
5. Kanner, L. (1943). Autistic disturbances of affective contact. *Nervous Child,* vol. 2, pp. 248 and 245, respectively. Retrieved from http://www.neurodiversity.com/library_kanner_1943.pdf.
6. Oller, J. W., and Oller, S. D. (2010). *Autism: The Diagnosis,*

Treatment, and Etiology of the Undeniable Epidemic. (Sudbury: Jones & Bartlett Publishers LLC, 2010), p. 49.

7. American Psychiatric Association (2013). *Diagnostic and Statistical Manual of Mental Disorders,* 5th Ed. *(DSM-5).* (Arlington: American Psychiatric Publishing, 2013), p. 53.

8. Blaxill, M. F. What's going on? The question of time trends in Autism. *Public Heath Reports,* Nov.-Dec. 2004, vol. 119, p. 548.

9. Centers for Disease Control and Prevention (2014). New data on autism spectrum disorder. Retrieved from http://www.cdc.gov/ncbddd/autism/data.html. It should be noted that the data published in 2014 are four years out of date and are undoubtedly underestimated. The data were derived from interviews of the parents or guardians of 8-year-olds living in 11 states within designated communities that were under CDC surveillance in 2010. See Centers for Disease Control and Prevention, *Morbidity and Mortality Weekly Report* (March 28, 2014), Prevalence of autism spectrum disorder among children aged 8 years—Autism and Developmental Disabilities Monitoring Network, 11 Sites, United States, 2010. Surveillance Summaries, vol. 63, no. 2, p. 6.

10. United States Government Accountability Office (GAO) (2014). Testimony Before the Subcommittee on Government Operations, Committee on Oversight and Government Reform, House of Representatives. Federal Autism Activities: Funding and Coordination Efforts, p. 1. Retrieved from http://www.gao.gov/assets/670/663313.pdf.

11. Autism Speaks (2012). New research finds annual cost of autism has more than tripled to $126 billion in the U.S. and reached £34 billion in the U.K. Retrieved from http://www.autismspeaks.org/about-us/press-releases/annual-cost-of-autism-triples.

12. Buescher, A. V., Cidav, Z., Knapp, M., and Mandell, D. S. (2014). Costs of autism spectrum disorders in the United Kingdom and the United States. *Journal of the American Medical Association Pediatrics.* doi:10.1001/jamapediatrics.2014.210 or 1 Aug. 2014, 168(8), p. 724.

13. Abramowicz, J. S., Fowlkes, J. B., Skelly, A. C., Stratmeyer, M. E., and Ziskin, M. C. (2008). Conclusions regarding epidemiology for obstetric ultrasound. *Journal of Ultrasound in Medicine,* vol. 27, no. 4, p. 641. In his "Epidemiology Primer" in this paper, Abramowicz states, "The

first point to consider in any analysis of a disease or a condition is its frequency. The two basic parameters are prevalence and incidence. Prevalence is the proportion of affected individuals at a specific point in time. It is obtained by dividing the total population into the number of affected individuals. Incidence is the frequency of new cases over a particular measure of time."

14. See McDonald, M. E., and Paul, J. F. (2010). U.S. Environmental Protection Agency, Timing of increased autistic disorder cumulative incidence. *Environmental Science & Technology,* vol. 44, no. 6, pp. 2114-15. This report found a dramatic increase in the cumulative incidence of autistic disorder (AD) beginning in the late 1980s "in the Danish, California, and worldwide data sets." The authors suggest (p. 2112) that "such an increase might be due to an increasing exposure to exogenous environmental factors (27, 29, 30) affecting susceptible individuals during vulnerable periods of their development."

15. Barclay, L. (2005), quoting Morton Ann Gernsbacher Ph.D., in Autism "epidemic"? A newsmaker interview with Morton Ann Gernsbacher, Ph.D., and Craig J. Newschaffer, Ph.D., p. 4. Retrieved from http://www.medscape.com/viewarticle/508429.

16. United States Government Accountability Office (2006). Federal Autism Activities: Funding for Research Has Increased, but Agencies Need to Resolve Surveillance Challenges, p. 3. Retrieved from http://www.gao.gov/new.items/d06700.pdf.

17. American Psychiatric Association. *Diagnostic and Statistical Manual of Mental Disorders*, 5th Ed. *(DSM-5)*. (Arlington: American Psychiatric Publishing, 2013), p. 58.

18. Yeargin-Allsopp, M. (2011). Workshop on U.S. Data to Evaluate Changes in the Prevalence of Autism Spectrum Disorders (ASDs), co-hosted by CDC and Autism Speaks, p. 7. Retrieved from http://www.cdc.gov/ncbddd/autism/documents/evaluatingchanges_workshopsummary.pdf.

19. U.S. Centers for Disease Control and Prevention (2012). Prevalence of Autism Spectrum Disorders—Autism and Developmental Disabilities Monitoring Network, 14 Sites, United States, 2008 – Surveillance Summaries, 30 March 2012, p. 2. Retrieved from http://

www.cdc.gov/mmwr/preview/mmwrhtml/ss6103a1.htm.

20. Centers for Disease Control and Prevention, National Center for Health Statistics, State and Local Area Integrated Telephone Survey 2011-2012 National Survey of Children's Health, p. 2. Retrieved from http://www.cdc.gov/nchs/slaits/nsch.htm.

21. Ibid.

22. Gallup, R. W., and Yazbak, F. E. (2007). When 1 in 150 is really 1 in 67. Retrieved from http://www.vaproject.org/yazbak/1-in-150-is-really-1-in-67-20071005.htm.

23. Ibid.

24. Centers for Disease Control and Prevention, *Morbidity and Mortality Weekly Report* (March 28, 2014). Prevalence of autism spectrum disorder among children aged 8 years—Autism and Developmental Disabilities Monitoring Network, 11 Sites, United States, 2010. Surveillance Summaries, vol. 63, no. 2, p. 2.

25. Ibid., p. 10.

26. Thomas Insel, M.D., director of The National Institute of Mental Health, writes in a 29 March 2012 article: "As diagnostic changes and ascertainment fail to explain the majority of the increase in autism prevalence, it seems prudent to assume that there are indeed more children affected. . . . Our working assumption is that there are both more children affected and more detected." The whys of increased prevalence. Retrieved from nimh.nih.gov/about/director/2012/autism-prevalence-more-affected-or-more-detected.shtml.

27. Currenti, S. A. (2010). Understanding and determining the etiology of autism. *Cellular and Molecular Neurobiology,* vol. 30, p. 161.

28. Muhle, R., Trentacoste, S. V., and Rapin, I. (2004). The genetics of autism. *Pediatrics,* May 2004, 113(5), Abstract. Retrieved from http://pediatrics.aappublications.org/content/113/5/e472.full.pdf.

29. Currenti, S. A. (2010). Understanding and determining the etiology of autism. *Cellular and Molecular Neurobiology*, vol. 30, p. 165.

30. Yazbak, F. E. (2013). Up, up and away: Autism in Boston schools. *Vaccination News,* 3 June 2013. Retrieved from http://www.vaccinationnews.com/2013-6-3-and-away-boston-schools-YazbakFE.

The article begins: "The title of a report in the 'Metro' section of the *Boston Globe* on May 29, 2013, was hard to miss: 'Boston Schools seek $6m more for special ed. Rise in students with autism helps prompt increase.'"

31. O'Brien, W. D. Jr. (1984). Safety of ultrasound with selective emphasis for obstetrics. *Seminars in Ultrasound, CT, and MRI*, vol. 5, no. 2, pp. 107-108. Retrieved from http://www.brl.uiuc.edu/Publications/1984/O'Brien-Ultrasound-105-1984.pdf.

32. Ibid., pp. 107-108.

33. Ibid., p. 108.

34. Miller, D. L. (2008). Safety assurance in obstetrical ultrasound. *Seminars in Ultrasound, CT and MRI,* vol. 29, p. 3. doi:10.1053/j.sult.2007.12.003.

35. O'Keeffe, D. F., and Abuhamad, A. (2013). Obstetric ultrasound utilization in the United States: Data from various health plans. *Seminars in Perinatology,* Oct. 2013; 37(5), Abstract. doi:10.1053/j.semperi.2013.06.003. Retrieved from http://www.ncbi/nim/nih.gov/pubmed/24176148.

36. Miller, D. L. (2008). Safety assurance in obstetrical ultrasound. *Seminars in Ultrasound, CT and MRI,* vol. 29, p. 3. doi:10.1053/j.sult.2007.12.003.

37. Whitworth, M., Bricker, L., Neilson, J. P., Dowswell, T. (2010). Cochrane Database of Systematic Reviews, published in the Cochrane Library 2010, issue 4, p. 2. Retrieved from http://www.update-software.com/BCP/WileyPDF/EN/CD007058.pdf.

38. Filly, R. A., and Crane, J. P. (2002). Routine obstetric sonography. *Journal of Ultrasound in Medicine,* vol. 21, no. 7, p. 2. Retrieved from http://www.jultrasoundmed.org/content/21/7/713.full.

39. Siddiqi, T. A. (2002). Medicine: Upper limits should be retained, in O'Brien, W. D. Jr., Abbott, J. G., Stratmeyer, M. E., Harris, G. R., Schafer, M. E., Siddiqi, T. A., Merritt, C. R. B., Duck, F. A., and Bendick, P. J. (2002). Acoustic output upper limits proposition: Should upper limits be retained? *Journal of Ultrasound in Medicine* 21, p. 1338-39.

40. Abramowicz, J. S. (2007). Prenatal exposure to ultrasound waves: Is there a risk? *Ultrasound in Obstetrics and Gynecology,* vol. 29, p. 366.

41. Barnett, S. B., Abramowicz, J. S., Ziskin, M. C., Maršál, K., and

Claudon, M. (2010). WFUMB Symposium on Safety of Nonmedical Use of Ultrasound. Ultrasound in Medicine and Biology, vol. 36, no. 8, p. 1210. doi:10.1016/j.ultrasoundbio.2010.04.005. Retrieved from http://www.wfumb.org/about/statements/nonmedicalUse.pdf.

42. Bioeffects and Safety Committee, International Society for Ultrasound in Obstetrics and Gynecology (J. Abramowicz, C. Brezinka, K. Salvesen and G. ter Haar), ISUOG statement on the non-medical use of ultrasound, 2009. *Ultrasound in Obstetrics and Gynecology,* vol. 33, p. 618.

43. Nicolson, M., and Fleming, J. E. E. (2013). *Imaging and Imagining the Fetus: The Development of Obstetric Ultrasound.* (Baltimore: The Johns Hopkins University Press, 2013), p. 232.

44. Blaxill, M. F. (2004). What's going on? The question of time trends in autism. Public Health Reports. Nov.-Dec. 2004, vol. 119, p. 536.

45. McDonald, M. E., and Paul, J. F. (2010). U.S. Environmental Protection Agency, Timing of increased autistic disorder cumulative incidence. *Environmental Science & Technology,* vol. 44, no. 6, p. 2112.

46. Currenti, S. A. (2010). Understanding and Determining the Etiology of Autism. *Cellular and Molecular Neurobiology*, vol. 30, p. 165.

47. Rodgers, C. (2012). Autism prevalence time trends, risk factors and prenatal ultrasound, p. 29. Presented to the Interagency Autism Coordinating Committee (IACC) on 10 July 2012. Retrieved from http://iacc.hhs.gov/events/2012/Slides_caroline_rodgers_071012.pdf.

48. Kurtz, A. B. (2003). The AIUM celebrates 50 years of excellence. *Journal of Ultrasound in Medicine,* vol. 22, no. 6, p. 545. Retrieved from http://www.jultrasoundmed.org/content/22/6/545.full.

49. Abramowicz, J. S. (2008). Bioeffects of obstetric ultrasound for the clinician: How to keep it safe, p. 5. Retrieved from https://iame.com/online/bioeffects_of_obstetric utlrasound/content.php.

50. Ibid.

II

Effects of Ultrasound on the Fetal Brain

There is ample published scientific evidence to demonstrate that exposure to diagnostic ultrasound can produce significant temperature increases in the fetal brain near bone.[1]

—Stanley B. Barnett, Ph.D.
in *The Safe Use of Ultrasound in Medicine and Biology (2012)*

The fetal brain and spinal cord, which form the central nervous system, are "sensitive to damage by physical agents, such as heat and ultrasound."[2] Autism is believed to originate with an injury to this highly sensitive neural tissue. Expectant parents should be aware that in 1992, changes in the FDA regulation of ultrasound allowed "delivery of almost eight times higher intensity into the fetal brain by ultrasound devices equipped with an approved ouput display."[3] Scientists have named ASD as a possible effect of ultrasound because experiments on embryonic animals have proved the fetal brain can be injured by ultrasound. The expectant mother should be informed of the risks when she asks, "Will this procedure harm the baby I am carrying?" Often this question is not even asked, so complete is the silence on the subject.[4] Prenatal ultrasound is entered into in blind trust. Society accepts the risks without knowing them, and seems to willfully ignore the epidemic of ASD associated with increasingly powerful ultrasound.

ASD Is a Result of Brain Injury Sustained in the Womb

ASD is believed to result from atypical brain development before birth.[5] When an ultrasound beam is focused on or near the unborn baby's head, it endangers the region of the brain that makes us human: the prefrontal cortex. This region of the brain, located behind the forehead, is the seat of creativity, personality, emotion, and the ability to reflect, conceptualize, and make associations. The moral qualities of a person, the knowledge of good and evil, lie in the prefrontal cortex. This area of the brain enables an individual to control his or her behavior, and if certain pathways are injured, behavior becomes erratic. Many symptoms of ASD—impairment in the capacity to empathize, enjoy shared experience, engage in reciprocal communication, understand social cues, and suppress rage—are attributable to defects in the prefrontal cortex.[6]

Expectant mothers may not realize that an ultrasound study of the head, face, and neck is one of the "minimal elements of a standard examination of fetal anatomy."[7] The brain and spinal column are exposed to ultrasound even in low-risk pregnancies. "Transabdominal sonography is the technique of choice to investigate the fetal CNS [central nervous system] during late first, second and third trimesters of gestation in low-risk pregnancies."[8] "Detailed evaluation of the fetal CNS *(fetal neurosonogram)* is also possible but requires specific expertise and sophisticated ultrasound machines."[9]

A Moderate Increase in Temperature May Cause Irreversible Brain Damage

Ultrasound is commonly perceived as noninvasive. However, it is an inescapable fact that as acoustic (ultrasound) energy passes through the fetus, it is absorbed by tissue and consequently generates heat, producing a rise in temperature.[10] This is called the *thermal* effect of ultrasound. Warming of fetal tissue, like fever in the newborn, is dangerous. "Among the various interactions between ultrasonic waves and biological tissues, a potential temperature rise is the most worrisome," writes Abramowicz.[11]

> **Biological tissues absorb ultrasound, *resulting in heating above normal physiological temperatures,* and an increase in temperature of sufficient magnitude and duration can damage or kill biological tissues. . . . *The effects of a moderate rise above normal physiological temperature can have important consequences for developing embryos or fetuses,* particularly if the central nervous system is involved. The actively dividing cells of the embryonic and fetal central nervous system are known to be highly susceptible to changes in temperature (Edwards, 1969b; Webster and Edwards, 1984; Shiota, 1982, 1988). *Interference with neural tissue is likely to have significant consequences on growth and development.*[12]**
> **[Emphasis added]**

"Data from animal studies demonstrate that exposure for 0.5 min. [30 seconds] to a temperature increase of 4°C [7.2° Fahrenheit] above the normal body temperature is potentially hazardous to embryonic and foetal development; exposures longer than 5 min. involves [sic] significant risk of harm."[13] Ultrasound causes a rapid rise in temperature, "with approximately 75% of the maximum heating occurring within 30 s [seconds]."[14] A typical ultrasound examination typically lasts 30 *minutes.* "Ziskin (44) reported that among 15,973 Doppler ultrasound examinations, the average duration was 27 minutes (and the longest 4 hours)."[15]

> **The physical mechanisms for bioeffects of ultrasound are generally separated into thermal and nonthermal. Heating by more than a few degrees above normal biological temperatures can perturb biological systems. . . . *At high intensities, rapid heating can cause simple cooking of tissue.*[16] [Emphasis added]**

Actively Dividing Brain Tissue Is Most Vulnerable

The developing brain is extremely susceptible to injury, or *insult.* It is particularly vulnerable to heat during the first trimester, according to Abramowicz.

> **This is a period of very high cell division (organogenesis). The brain appears to be the most susceptible organ. The early stages of embryogenesis have been shown in mammals to be especially sensitive to heat in terms of induction of birth defects. Current commercially available diagnostic ultrasound scanners are capable of achieving the levels of tissue temperature increase shown in a related mammalian system under carefully controlled experimental conditions to cause deleterious effects.**[17]

Developing bone has a much greater capacity to absorb heat than other fetal tissue. "The absorption coefficient of bone may be as much as 50 times greater than most soft tissue."[18] The frontal cortex is particularly vulnerable to heat because it lies close to the frontal bone.

> **[F]rom a safety perspective, the tissue that has the greatest potential for bio-effects from ultrasound-induced heating is bone, or developing bone. . . . Tissues lying close to, or in contact with, bone are also at risk of heating by conduction from the bone. . . . As actively dividing cells are most susceptible to damage by heat, the foetal cerebral cortex, situated close to the skull bone, is at risk of damage by ultrasound-induced temperature increase.**[19]

Proof of Ultrasound-Induced Disruption of Fetal Brain Development

During pregnancy, the architecture of the human brain develops according to a definite pattern and a "precise schedule."[20] Brain cells (neurons) originate in the cerebral cortex and travel, or migrate, to the place where they will serve their intended purpose. Any disruption of this process, called neuronal migration, will have a profound effect on the development of the individual. In a discussion of animal experiments on the effects of hyperthermia, Church and Barnett stated: "In embryonic development a lapse of a few hours can lead to substantial delay or disturbance in neurological development."[21]

When the ultrasound beam is focused on or near the human brain—either during cranial studies or simply to capture an image of the face—the trajectory of neurodevelopment can be altered. A landmark 2006 study led by Pasko Rakic, M.D., Ph.D., the prominent neuroscientist who heads the Rakic Lab at Yale University Medical School,[22] proved frequent and excessive use of prenatal ultrasound could alter the development of the mammalian brain by preventing neurons from reaching their appropriate place in the brain structure. The study, "Prenatal Exposure to Ultrasound Waves Impacts Neuronal Migration in Mice," was the first to test "the rate of migration in the cerebral cortex" of mice and chemically tag brain cells in order to follow their migration. A small but significant number of cells became "lost" and could not serve their intended function. These anatomical changes were observable under the microscope. The research team reported:

> **Neurons of the cerebral neocortex in mammals, including humans, are generated during fetal life**

> **in the proliferative zones and then migrate to their final destinations by following an inside-to-outside sequence. . . . Our analysis of over 335 animals reveals that, when exposed to USW [ultrasound waves] for a total of 30 min. or longer during the period of their migration, a small but statistically significant number of neurons fail to acquire their proper position and remain scattered within inappropriate cortical layers and/or in the subjacent white matter.**[23]

Rakic's widely publicized experiment, whose express purpose was to prove that excessive use of prenatal ultrasound should be avoided, was interpreted as a warning of the risks to the human fetus. The authors stated: "[O]ur results in pregnant mice support the recommendations by the Food and Drug Administration that warn against the use of medically nonindicated or commercial prenatal ultrasound videos."[24] "The technical rigor of this study, which comes from a laboratory that generated much of our understanding of normal cortical development, has to be taken seriously," stated one physician in an interview with *Neurology Today*, adding that "if there was ever any scientific proof needed to halt the expansion of recreational ultrasound, this study provides it."[25]

Britain's Health Protection Agency wrote in 2010:

> **The results of this study in mice are important because there is the possibility that qualitatively similar effects could occur in humans: the same tissues in different species tend to exhibit the same acoustic properties, suggesting the same interactions will occur. However, direct extrapolation to humans is problematic, as recognized by Ang et al (2006), due in part to the obvious differences that exist between the developing cerebral cortex in rodents and humans in terms of**

numbers of neurons and the time and complexity of their migratory processes. This limitation applies to all studies using animal models.[26]

The American Institute of Ultrasound in Medicine (AIUM) Bioeffects Committee criticized the 2006 study.[27] Nevertheless, the value of the experiment lies in its proof that prenatal ultrasound can alter brain development in mammals, producing subtle differences between unexposed and exposed animals. Ang, *et al.*, stated that earlier evidence of the effects of prenatal ultrasound in animals had prompted their study. "It has been reported that the exposure of pregnant mice and non-human primates to USW may affect the behavior of their exposed offspring (26, 27)," they wrote. "There also is some evidence that the frequent exposure of the human fetus to USW is associated with a decrease in newborn body weight (28, 29), an increase in the frequency of left-handedness (30), and delayed speech (31). In addition, it was reported that diagnostic levels of ultrasound can disrupt membrane attachments or cells both *in vitro* (32, 33) [in the test tube] and in vivo (34) [in living tissue] and alter the cell cycle of the intestinal epithelium *in vivo* (35). Because ultrasound energy is a high-frequency mechanical vibration (36), we hypothesized that it might influence membrane-mediated, cell-to-cell attachments and/or nuclear translocation essential for neuronal migration."[28]

In the scientific literature, the disruption of neuronal migration is cited as a possible cause of autism and other neurodevelopmental disorders:

> **Disruption or even slowing down of neuronal migration may result not only in gross and obvious but also *subtle abnormalities* in neuronal positioning that indirectly affect the pattern of synaptic circuits**

Project Information -- NIH RePORTER -- NIH Research Portfolio Online Reporting Tools Expenditures and Results

U.S. Department of Health & Human Services

NIH **Research Portfolio Online Reporting Tools**
(RePORT)

QUICK LINKS RESEARCH ORGANIZATIONS WORKFORCE

Home > RePORTER > Project Information

Project Information

5R01NS01481-32

DESCRIPTION DETAILS RESULTS HISTORY SUBPROJECTS SIMILAR PROJECTS NEARBY PROJECTS BETA LINKS

Project Number:	5R01NS01481-32	**Contact PI / Project Leader:**	**RAKIC, PASKO**
Title:	NEUROGENETIC PROCESSES IN THE FETAL BRAIN	**Awardee Organization:**	**YALE UNIVERSITY**

Total project funding amount for 34 projects is $9,312,696*

Only NIH and CDC funding data for fiscal years 2000 and later are available.

Yale University's Rakic Lab received a grant for $9,312,696 for studies to include the effects of prenatal ultrasound on macaque monkeys. The results are anticipated in 2015. This image represents the top portion of the first page of the document.

> **(Algan and Rakic, 1997; Ang et al., 2006). . . . [I]n many cases the neuronal malpositioning *may be subtle and cannot be detected readily* by conventional histopathologic techniques. Such misplaced neurons may be involved in a variety of idiopathic neurological disorders that range from childhood epilepsy and mental retardation to autism and developmental dyslexia. . . . In conclusion, the identity, synpatic relationship and, ultimately, function of neurons in the brain depends on their proper location, which is achieved by long distance migration in the embryonic brain.[29] [Emphasis added]**

Following the 2006 study, Yale's Rakic Lab received a $9,312,696 grant from the National Institutes of Health for projects to include research on the effects of prenatal ultrasound in the macaque monkey, whose brain is more comparable to that of humans than the mouse brain. (See opposite page.) In the project description, "neuronal misplacement" was linked with "the recent increase in incidence" of autism and other developmental disorders:

> **A major emphasis will be on the possible effect of ultrasound on neuronal migration rate and placement in both murine and primate cerebral cortex, as this study may have important biomedical implications. Emphasis on the early aspects of neuronal production and proper placement in mammalian species will provide new insight into the pathogenesis of genetic and acquired cortical malformations affecting higher brain function. . . . *The proposed studies are even more pressing given the recent increase in incidence of developmental disorders of higher brain functions such as autism,* childhood epilepsy, developmental**

dyslexia and mental retardation, possibly attributable to neuronal misplacement during formation of the cerebral cortex.[30] [Emphasis added]

The anticipated completion date of the Rakic Lab's project, including study of the effects of prenatal ultrasound on macaque monkeys, is January 31, 2015. NIH did not respond to this author's written requests for any results to date.

Manuel Casanova, M.D., states there is evidence of cell displacement in autistic individuals. In an interview he discussed this evidence in layman's terms:

[W]hatever is happening in autism is a reflection of a brain dysfunction. It's not a reflection of a mind dysfunction; this has a physical basis. . . . In the brains of autistic individuals you actually find cells where they shouldn't be, and those cells tie themselves together; they create new circuitry and in many cases are the basis for seizures. The interesting thing about this finding is that it will vary from one patient to the next. Whenever you see these so-called heterotopias—cell displacement—it may happen at the front of the brain for one patient, at the back of the brain for another; it may actually happen outside the hemispheres in a place we call the cerebellum. . . . So every single patient is actually different.[31]

In a scientific paper on the effects of prenatal ultrasound in relation to autism, Casanova and E. L. Williams discuss the remarkable *heterogeneity* of the autism spectrum: the symptoms of autism vary widely from person to person. Their theory helps explain why ASD takes different forms:

> **While the concept of autism as a spectrum has been generally well accepted by professional and lay communities alike, in spite of the spectrum's commonalities the heterogeneity of the condition is undeniable . . . even individuals falling under the same diagnostic label exhibit not only behavioral but genetic (103) and neuroanatomical and physiological hetereogeneity (20). A uniting factor when considering this diversity may be the action of certain teratogens, such as ultrasound, and the distinct effects they have based on timing, number, and strength of exposure. Also, the diverse heterotopias observed in autism may be explained by timing of exposure and the distinct effects it has on cellular proliferation, differentiation, and migration.**[32]

The paper cited above begins with a reference to autism in Casanova's family:

> **"Would you like to see a picture of your baby?"**
> — *The first words uttered by an obstetrician to my daughter at 12 weeks of gestation.*

The Dearth of Valid Scientific Research

Assurances of safety proffered to expectant mothers should be founded on the bedrock of scientific evidence. In reality, no valid studies of the bioeffects of prenatal ultrasound have been conducted at the higher intensities allowed since 1992. Abramowicz states, with his own emphasis:

> **[I]t must once more be stressed that there has been *no* epidemiological study published on populations**

> **scanned after 1992, when regulations were altered and acoustic output of diagnostic instruments permitted to reach levels many times higher than previously allowed.**[33]

The misleading portrayal of ultrasound's "exemplary safety record" is based primarily on studies that scientists themselves have invalidated. First, most existing studies were conducted with pre-1992 equipment, before the maximum power of ultrasound machines increased nearly eightfold. Second, most studies suffer from "extremely low statistical power," "a low follow-up rate; no unexposed group for comparison; no indication of gestational age at time of exposure; no indication of the number of exposures or the type of ultrasound exposure (pulse-echo or Doppler or both),"[34] and give no indication of the reason for the procedure, the name of the manufacturer, the model number of the ultrasound equipment used, or the number of examinations. Yet, this body of research—with its outdated equipment, unscientific methodology, and failure to account for safety lapses—is the basis for upholding the safety of routine prenatal ultrasound.

> **The absence of reported effects stem largely from the fact that subtle effects have not been studied at all.**[35]

> **[T]he lack of findings is just that. It does not "prove" safety. Subtle behavioral or psychological changes would be extremely difficult to show.**[36]

> **Diagnostic ultrasound is assumed to be safe. This opinion is supported by a general lack of independently confirmed adverse effects from ultrasound exposure in mothers or children. However, these conclusions have limited relevance to the way ultrasound is**

currently used in medicine. For example, there are no epidemiological data relevant to the increased acoustic outputs available with modern equipment. . . .[37]

[W]hether diagnostic ultrasound has induced or can induce harmful effects is not established. Harmful effects have not been shown so far, which means only that.[38]

ASD Is a "Subtle" Effect of Prenatal Ultrasound

Abramowicz states that although, "as far as we know, ultrasound will not induce major abnormalities, such as limb reductions or central nervous system gross anomalies, *the possibility of subtle effects cannot be ruled out.* These are, unfortunately, very difficult to demonstrate. [Emphasis added.]"[39]

To understand why physicians and scientists have "missed" the bioeffects of prenatal ultrasound, it is important to know the medical definition of the word *subtle.* The defect that causes symptoms of autism may be infinitesimal, in contrast to obvious or gross effects that can be readily identified. In some cases ASD may not be diagnosed until the individual encounters a situation that taxes the impaired brain. The brain does not reach full maturity until around age 25, and subtle alterations may be overlooked.

O'Brien cautions that we should not conclude ultrasound is safe without further laboratory studies. He refers to the fact that ionizing radiation, including x-rays, was once considered harmless:

Diagnostic medicine has generated an enormity of clinical experience with ultrasound. During this time, it is extremely encouraging that no deleterious clinical effects

have been reported. However, one must be cautious to conclude from this experiential data base that ultrasound can be thought of as safe. There is no substitute for carefully derived scientific findings. One only needs to examine the history of ionizing radiation and other chemical and physical agents to realize that many subtle effects would not have been discovered without comprehensive experimental studies using animals.[40] [Emphasis added]

No matter how many laboratory experiments show a lack of effect from diagnostic ultrasound, it will always be necessary to study directly its effect in human populations before any definitive statement regarding risk can be made.[41]

[I]t must be emphasized that neither theoretic calculations nor experimental results can yield unambiguous and definite evidence that fully guarantees the safety of ultrasound diagnostics, particularly in regards to delayed, subtle effects. Such effects would be very difficult to detect, given that the incidence of congenital anomalies in the general population is about 3%.[42]

In an early paper O'Brien poses the questions that remain for all who would administer or undergo prenatal ultrasound:

The use of diagnostic ultrasound in the clinical practice of medicine is generally recognized as not representing any hazard. Whereas agents such as drugs are generally not considered safe until proven so, radiation, such as ultrasound, is generally considered safe until proven otherwise. The studies necessary to assess the risk

associated with human exposure to ultrasound have not been done. It is, however, important to recognize that ultrasound at sufficient energy levels is capable of totally destroying biological tissues. <u>Thus the question of risk becomes (1) what biological systems are most sensitive to ultrasound and (2) what exposure levels impose a significant risk on those systems</u>?[43] (Emphasis added)

In answer to the first question, scientists state that the central nervous system—the brain and spinal cord—are the fetal organs most sensitive to ultrasound. They cannot answer the second question with certainty. Ultrasound physicist Francis A. Duck, Ph.D., states, "It remains an open question what threshold and of what acoustic quantity is sufficient to result in any transient or permanent disturbance to the embryological structure."[44]

> **The susceptibility of an embryo or fetus to a physical or chemical agent is strongly determined by its stage of development. . . . [T]he development from a zygote to a full-term fetus is the dynamic interaction of many systems working in unison. Any agent or insult that disrupts the normal developmental program could potentially jeopardize normal intrauterine development. Because the very young embryo consists of a limited number of cells, the introduction of a physical or chemical agent at this stage of gestation could have a major impact on development.**[45]

This chapter has presented overwhelming evidence that ultrasound is capable of damaging the fetal brain. If any question remains, this author would propose a study of the effects of ultrasound on embryonic pigs, whose neurological development is similar to that of humans. Medical history has shown it is not always prudent to wait for studies. Since there is no cure for ASD, and human studies cannot be performed, the wisest course is prevention. Under no circumstances should the ultrasound beam be directed at the fetal brain. It must be remembered, however, that all organ systems of the unborn child are vulnerable to ultrasound:

> **Potential direct fetal effects from ultrasound are of special concern because the fetus often receives whole body exposure during diagnostic imaging. . . . Many fetal systems, such as the neural, visual, endocrine, behavioral and reproductive systems, are immature at birth and development continues well into adolescence.**[46]

It is this author's belief that every child exposed to prenatal ultrasound is diminished in ways we have only begun to understand.

ENDNOTES

II. Effects of Ultrasound on the Fetal Brain

1. Barnett, S. B. (2001). Intracranial temperature elevation from diagnostic ultrasound. *Ultrasound in Medicine and Biology*, vol. 27, no. 7, p. 884.

2. Barnett, S. B. (2001). Intracranial temperature elevation from diagnostic ultrasound. *Ultrasound in Medicine and Biology* (2001), vol. 27, no. 7, p. 883, Abstract.

3. Ibid. The complete passage reads: "Recent changes in the FDA regulation allow delivery of almost eight times higher intensity into the fetal brain by ultrasound devices that incorporate an approved real-time output display in their design."

4. Science writer Caroline Rodgers refers to the silence surrounding the connection between prenatal ultrasound and autism in her 2010 work, "The Elephant in the Room," presented at the 22 Oct. 2010 meeting of the Interagency Autism Coordinating Committee. Rodgers sets forth a logical argument implicating prenatal ultrasound in the autism epidemic. Retrieved from http://iacc.hhs.gov/events/2010/slides_caroline_rodgers_102210.pdf.

5. "During the past two decades, neuroimaging and autopsy studies have revealed a variety of developmental brain abnormalities, all implicating that the etiologic insult likely occurs during early prenatal development (61, 62)." American Academy of Pediatrics – Committee on Children with Disabilities (2001). Technical Report: The Pediatrician's Role in the Diagnosis and Management of Autism Spectrum Disorder in Children." *Pediatrics,* vol. 107, no. 5, p. 4. Retrieved from http://www.pediatrics.org/cgi/content/full/107/5/e85.

6. The author suggests that the increasing incidence of bizarre shootings by young people—such as those in Aurora and Columbine, Colorado, and at Sandy Hook Elementary School in Newtown, Connecticut, followed by similar events—may be attributable to individuals with severe damage to the prefrontal cortex as a result of excessive sonography during pregnancy.

7. ACR-ACOG-AIUM-SRU Practice parameter for the

performance of obstetrical ultrasound (2013), p. 9. Retrieved from http://www.acr.org/Quality-Safety/Standards-Guidelines/Practice-Guidelines-by-Modality/Ultrasound. Click on title.

8. Sonographic examination of the fetal central nervous system: Guidelines for performing the "basic examination" and the "fetal neurosonogram" (2007), vol. 29, p. 110. *Ultrasound in Obstetrics and Gynecology,* 29:109-116. doi:0.1002/uog.3909.

9. Ibid., p. 109.

10. Sheiner, E., Shoham-Vardi, I., Pombar, X., Hussey, M. J., Strassner, H. T., and Abramowicz, J. S. (2007). An increased thermal index can be achieved when performing Doppler studies in obstetric sonography. *Journal of Ultrasound in Medicine,* vol. 26, p. 72. The authors continue: "The thermal indices (TIS) express the potential for rise in temperature along the ultrasound's beam." Retrieved from jultrasoundmed.org/content/26/1/71.full.pdf.

11. Abramowicz, J. S. (2002). Ultrasound in obstetrics and gynecology: Is this hot technology too hot? *Journal of Ultrasound in Medicine,* vol. 21, no. 12, p. 1329.

12. Church, C. C., and Barnett, S. B. (2013). Ultrasound-induced heating and its biological consequences, in ter Haar (ed.), *The Safe Use of Ultrasound in Medical Diagnosis,* p. 47. Retrieved from http://www.birjournals.org/site/book/Safe_Use_of_Ultrasound.pdf.

13. Church, C. C., and Barnett, S. B. (2012). Ultrasound-induced heating and its biological consequences, in *The Safe Use of Ultrasound in Medical Diagnosis,* p. 63.

14. Barnett, S. B. (2001). Intracranial temperature elevation from diagnostic ultrasound. *Ultrasound in Medicine and Biology,* vol. 27, no. 7, p. 883.

15. Abramowicz, J. S., Barnett, S. B., Duck, F. A., Edmonds, P. D., Hynynen, K., and Ziskin, M.C. (2008). Fetal thermal effects of diagnostic ultrasound. *Journal of Ultrasound in Medicine,* vol. 27, no. 4, p. 544.

16. Stratmeyer, M. C., Greenleaf, J. F., Dalecki, D., and Salvesen, K. (2008). Fetal ultrasound: Mechanical effects. *Journal of Ultrasound in Medicine,* vol. 27, no. 4, p 2. Retrieved from http://www.jultrasoundmed.org/content/27/4/597.long.

17. Abramowicz, J. S. (2002). Ultrasound in obstetrics and

gynecology: Is this hot technology too hot? *Journal of Ultrasound in Medicine,* vol. 21, no. 12, p. 3.

18. Church, C. C., and Barnett, S. B. (2012). Ultrasound-induced heating and its biological consequences, in *The Safe Use of Ultrasound in Medical Diagnosis,* p. 48.

19. Church, C. C., and Barnett, S. B. (2012). Ultrasound-induced heating and its biological consequences, in *The Safe Use of Ultrasound in Medical Diagnosis,* p. 49.

20. Ang, ESBC Jr., Gluncic, V., Duque, A., Schafer, M. E., and Rakic, P. (2006). Prenatal exposure to ultrasound waves impacts neuronal migration in mice. Proceedings of the National Academy of Sciences of the United States of America, vol. 103, no. 34, p. 12903. Retrieved from http://www.pnas.org/cgi/doi/10.1073/pnas.0605294103.

21. Church, C. C., and Barnett, S. B. (2012). Ultrasound-induced heating and its biological consequences, in *The Safe Use of Ultrasound in Medical Diagnosis,* p. 52.

22. Rakic, formerly a neurosurgeon, is currently the Duberg Professor of Neurobiology and Neurology, chair of the Department of Neurobiology, and director of the Kavli Intsitute of Neuroscience. In 2008 he was awarded the first Kavli Prize in Neuroscience in honor of his three decades of pioneering anatomical studies "that revealed how neurons in the developing cerebral cortex are generated and how they assemble themselves into highly ordered, distinctively layered, and densely interconnected circuits that direct higher order sensory and motor functions," according to the 28 May 2008 *Yale News.* The $3-million mouse study was funded by the National Institute of Neurological Disorders and Stroke of the National Institutes of Health.

23. Ang, ESBC Jr., Gluncic, V., Duque, A., Schafer, M. E, and Rakic, P. (2006) Prenatal exposure to ultrasound waves impacts neuronal migration in mice. Proceedings of the National Academy of Sciences of the United States of America, vol. 103, no. 34, p. 12903. Retrieved from http://www.pnas.org/cgi/doi/10.1073/pnas.0605294103.

24. Ibid., p. 12908.

25. Samson, K. (2006). Prolonged ultrasound disrupts brain development in fetal mice. *Neurology Today,* vol. 6, issue 18,

p. 2. Retrieved from http://journals.lww.com/neurotodayonline/Fulltext/2006/09190/Prolonged_ultrasound_Disrupts_Brain_Development_ir.2.aspx.

26. Health Protection Agency (2010). Health effects of exposure to ultrasound and infrasound (2010). *Report of the Independent Advisory Group on Non-ionizing Radiation,* p. 104. Retrieved from http://www.hpa.org.uk/webc/HPAWebFile/HPAweb_C/1265028759369.

27. American Institute of Ultrasound in Medicine (AIUM) (2009), Bioeffects Literature Review: Prenatal Exposure to Ultrasound Waves Impacts Neuronal Migration in Mice. *Journal of Ultrasound in Medicine,* vol. 28, pp. 558-561. AIUM's criticism included the following statements: "The reported effects on neuronal migration were not observed at clinically relevant exposures;" "The statistical analysis is inappropriate, and internal replication of the data is incomplete;" and "too few animals were used."

28. Ang, ESBC Jr., Gluncic, V., Duque, A., Schafer, M. E., and Rakic, P. (2006). Prenatal exposure to ultrasound waves impacts neuronal migration in mice. Proceedings of the National Academy of Sciences of the United States of America, vol. 103, no. 34, p. 12903. Retrieved from http://www.pnas.org/cgi/doi/10.1073/pnas.0605294103.

29. Metin, C., Vallee, R. B., Rakic, P., and Bhide, P. G. (2008). Modes and mishaps of neuronal migration in the mammalian brain. *Journal of Neuroscience*, vol. 28(46), p. 11750. doi:10.1523/JNeurosci.3860-08.2008.

30. NIH Awards by Location and Organization. Retrieved from http://report.nih.gov/award/index.cfm?view=orgdetail&orgid=9420201&ot=MS&fy=2004&state=CT&ic=NINDS&fm=&page=1. This document is difficult to access. See http://grantome.com/grant/NIH/R01-NS014841-35.

31. Casanova, M. (2011). Transcription of online audio interview with Rob Sidell. Interview with Dr. Casanova—Does ultrasound contribute to ASD? Autism International Association. Retrieved from http://www.autismone.org/content/interview-dr-casanova-does-ultrasound-contribute-asd.

32. Williams, E. L., and Casanova, M. F. (2010), Potential teratogenic effects of ultrasound on corticogenesis: Implications for autism. *Medical Hypotheses.* doi:10.1016.j.mehy.2010.01.027, p. 4.

33. Abramowicz, J. C. (2001). Bioeffects of obstetric ultrasound for the clinician: How to keep it safe, p. 6. Institute for Medical Education. Retrieved from https://iame.com/online/bioeffects_of_obstetric_ultrasound/content.php.

34. Stratmeyer, M. E., and Fisher, B. R. Exposure to medical ultrasound: Studies of human effects, in Repacholi, M. H., Grandolfo, M., and Rindi, A. (eds.), *Ultrasound: Medical Applications, Biological Effects, and Hazard Potential* (New York and London: Plenum Press, 1986, reissued 2013), pp. 220-224.

35. Duck, F. A. (1999). Is it safe to use diagnostic ultrasound during the first trimester? *Ultrasound in Obstetrics and Gynecology,* vol. 13, p. 387.

36. Abramowicz, J. S., Barnett, S. B., Duck, F. A., Edmonds, P. D., Hynynen, K. H., and Ziskin, M. C. Fetal thermal effects of diagnostic ultrasound. *Journal of Ultrasound in Medicine,* vol. 27, no. 4, p. 553.

37. Church, C. C., and Barnett, S. B. (2012). Ultrasound-induced heating and its biological consequences, in *The Safe Use of Ultrasound in Medical Diagnosis,* p. 47.

38. Abramowicz, Jacques S. (2002). Ultrasound in obstetrics and gynecology: Is this hot technology too hot? *Journal of Ultrasound in Medicine* 21:12, p. 5.

39. Abramowicz, J. S. (2012). Fetal Doppler: How to keep it safe? *Clinical Obstetrics and Gynecology,* vol. 53, no. 4, p. 843.

40. O'Brien, W. D. (1998). Assessing the risks for modern diagnostic ultrasound imaging, p. 2. Retrieved from http://www.brl.uiuc.edu/Projects/Bioeffects/Assesssing.php.

41. Ziskin, M. C., and Petitti, D. B. (1988). Epidemiology of human exposure to ultrasound: A critical review. *Ultrasound in Medicine and Biology,* vol. 14, no. 2, p. 91.

42. Abramowicz, J. S. (2008). Bioeffects of obstetric ultrasound for the clinician: How to keep it safe, p. 9. Retrieved from https://iame.com/online/bioeffects_of_obstetric_ultrasound/content.php.

43. O'Brien, W. D. Jr. Medical Physics Monograph No. 6, in Fullerton, G. D., and Zagzebski, J. A. (eds.), *Medical Physics of CT and*

Ultrasound: Tissue Imaging and Characterization (Madison: Medical Physics Publishing, 1980), p. 578.

44. Duck, F. A. (1999). Editorial: Is it safe to use diagnostic ultrasound during the first trimester? *Ultrasound in Obstetrics and Gynecology,* vol. 13, p. 387.

45. Fisher, B. R., and Stratmeyer, M. D. Developmental and teratogenic effects of ultrasound, in *Ultrasound: Medical Applications, Biological Effects, and Hazard Potential* (New York and London: Plenum Press, 1986, reissued 2013), p. 196.

46. Ibid., p. 197.

III
The "Uncharted Waters" of Ultrasound Safety

***The use of ultrasound without a medical indication to view the fetus, obtain images of the fetus or determine the fetal gender is inappropriate and contrary to responsible medical practice.*[1]**

—American Institute of Ultrasound in Medicine, 2012

This safety guideline, published by one of the world's foremost organizations for the safety of ultrasound, means that ultrasound is a medical procedure to be used in the diagnosis of suspected fetal abnormalities. It poses a risk to the fetus, and there is no justification for taking that risk without a valid medical reason[2] and without the prospect of medical benefit to the unborn child. Despite this recommendation of the American Institute for Ultrasound in Medicine and other world organizations, prenatal ultrasound is used with excessive frequency for no particular cause, at increasing intensity without adequate safety controls, and earlier in gestation, when the developing central nervous system is considered most sensitive. For decades, the *assumption* of absolute safety has allowed this practice to proliferate beyond its intended purpose and beyond scientists' ability to assure its safety.

Advances in ultrasound technology have brought "not only increased diagnostic capabilities, but also uncharted waters as far as safety considerations are concerned,"[3] writes Gail ter Haar, Ph.D., in her preface to the 2012 book *The Safe Use of Ultrasound in Medical Diagnosis*, written by international experts in ultrasound safety. She states, "What is evident from the information presented in this book is that there are many gaps in our knowledge about ultrasound safety."[4]

Around the world, expectant mothers typically receive a simplified version of AIUM's official safety statement "Conclusions Regarding Epidemiology for Obstetric Ultrasound," which begins: "Based on the epidemiological data available and on current knowledge of interactive mechanisms, there is insufficient justification to warrant a conclusion of a causal relationship between diagnostic ultrasound and recognized adverse effects in humans."[5] The following language appears under "Risks" in a brochure prepared by the Mayo Clinic: "Routine fetal ultrasounds are considered safe for both mother and baby. Researchers haven't noted any adverse effects of fetal ultrasounds in children followed for several years after birth."[6] A 2008 publication of Kaiser Permanente, later revised, stated, "Ultrasound uses harmless sound waves that are directed at organs in the body. The sound waves used in ultrasound exams have been safely used for many years."[7]

In the scientific literature, scientists are careful to qualify their assertions of safety:

> **[E]xperimental evidence suggests that the interaction of ultrasound with developing biological systems is not fully understood. . . . Of concern are the subtle and/or long-term manifestations of frequent intrauterine exposure, particularly when considering those areas of the fetus that develop throughout gestation such as the brain and bone. . . .[8]**

> **While it seems evident that DUS [diagnostic ultrasound] does not cause major structural/anatomic anomalies in the fetuses being scanned, more subtle effects cannot completely be ruled out and certain steps are recommended for the clinical end-user to assure safety.[9]**

[D]iagnostic ultrasound can only be considered safe if used prudently. Ultrasound examinations should only be performed by competent personnel who are trained and updated in safety matters. It is also important that ultrasound devices are appropriately maintained.[10]

[T]he lack of recent epidemiological research and human data in the field is appalling, as is the lack of knowledge of the end users.[11]

FDA Regulation Places Ultrasound Safety in the Hands of the Operator

Expectant mothers should be aware of the consequences of the FDA's regulatory decision of 1992, which has been debated extensively in the scientific literature.

During the early 1990s the FDA allowed an almost eightfold increase in the maximum intensity (acoustic output) of ultrasound machines used in obstetrics, "including first-trimester scanning. No epidemiological or other evidence was then, or is now, available to support the assertion of safety at these higher exposures."[12]

This step had two important consequences: a beam of higher intensity carried an increased risk to the fetus,[13] and at the same time safety became the ultimate responsibility of the operator, who was expected to complete an FDA-recommended education program but was not required to be credentialed.

In giving users the capability "to operate their systems at levels much higher than previously had been possible," the FDA recognized that "the possibility existed for the potential to do harm to the patient."[14] It agreed to relax the upper limits of acoustic intensity upon condition that the manufacturer of the ultrasound device install two on-screen safety indices, the thermal index (TI) and the mechanical index (MI). These were intended to register the acoustic output, or power levels, and enable the operator to minimize exposure. During the exam, the numerical indices give the operator "information about the potential for temperature increase (the Thermal Index) and mechanical damage (the Mechanical Index)."[15] TI and MI represent the two main types of physical harm known to result from ultrasound: (1) effects associated with a rise in temperature and (2) nonthermal bioeffects, such as cavitation.[16] The "so-called 'safety indices'"[17]—as Duck calls them—are crude estimates of risk and serve only as a guide.

The Output Display Standard (ODS), which regulated use of the new equipment features, was implemented in 1992. "A very important aspect of the implementation of the ODS as explicitly emphasized in the original recommendations for adoption was education of the end users about bioeffects of ultrasound and safety-related issues," writes Abramowicz.[18] In order to obtain FDA approval of the more powerful equipment, manufacturers were required to provide an educational program designed to guide operators in following the principle of ALARA, whose "intent is to obtain needed diagnostic information with minimum risk to the patient."[19] The initials stand for As Low As Reasonably Achievable. "This principle holds that the goal of a study is not an image with the maximal quality achievable but one that is sufficient to make a diagnostic judgment with the least possible exposure."[20] An operator must be highly educated to conduct a prenatal ultrasound exam in accordance with ALARA.

The following excerpts indicate the sophistication of the topics to be covered in educational materials supplied by the manufacturer.

3.4 Track 3 – Education Program for the Clinical End-User

3.4.1 ALARA Education Program

3.4.2.2 Thermal Mechanisms.

You should provide the following:

· description of thermal bioeffects—temperature rise;
· tissue type (soft, bone, fluid) and relative aborption;
· transducer type (frequency, focusing) and relationship to exposure;
· attenuation, absorption, and scattering mechanisms in different tissue types; and
· spatial volume of insonified tissue (at focus, or elsewhere), including:
  · homogeneity of tissue in insonified volume (effects of layering);
  · soft tissue;
  · bone tissue (fetal, skull, other); and
  · fluids, gas.

3.4.2.3 Nonthermal Mechanisms

You should provide the following:

· description of mechanical effects—cavitation and role of bubbles;
· factors that produce cavitation, including:
  · pressure (compressional, rarefactional);
  · frequency;
  · beam focusing;
  · pulsed/continuous;
  · standing waves;
  · boundaries; and
  · type of material and ambient conditions.
· types of cavitation, including:

    - **stable and inertial cavitation;**
    - **microstreaming; and**
    - **nucleation sites.**
- **threshold phenomena for different types of tissues; and**
- **bioeffects data on animals (lung hemorrhage, intestinal hemorrhage).**[21]

It is clear that the ALARA guidelines for prudent use of fetal ultrasound require an understanding of the biology and physics of ultrasound exposure. However, the FDA has not enforced the education of clinical users, and operator error presents a serious risk. In 2007 Abramowicz co-authored a study that reported in Europe and the United States, "approximately 70% of clinicians (physicians, sonographers, and nurses who perform ultrasound) . . . do not know what TI and MI represent and do not even know that these appear on-screen during clinical ultrasound examinations."[22] A survey of European obstetricians, gynecologists, and "internationally recognized experts in fetal ultrasound" revealed that most respondents had "very poor knowledge of ultrasound," Maršál observed. He commented: "It can be presumed that . . . [a]mong non-professionals that use fetal ultrasound for non-medical commercial purposes, no understanding of the safety issues whatsoever can be expected."[23]

Gaps in Knowledge and Safety

There is currently no consistent method of defining a "dose" of ultrasound. Unable to systematically control the dose, the operator will at times exceed safe dosage. The on-screen safety indices do not take exposure time into account. If the operator cannot determine how long the ultrasound beam dwells on a given part of the fetus, it is difficult to judge when it would be prudent to halt the ultrasound exam.

Comparing x-ray with ultrasound, Duck states, "there is very little equivalent investment in the measure of exposure to ultrasound," and "the concept of dose has still to be properly developed":

> **The measurement of radiation is central to the safe and effective management of radiological imaging. . . . [O]bstetrics established ultrasound as a preferred safe modality, substantially replacing the use of X-ray imaging with its known hazard. Nevertheless, ultrasound examinations do expose the patient to external radiation, albeit associated with different hazards than those from ionizing radiation.**[24]

Ter Haar frames the issue of dose by comparing x-ray, which emits ionizing radiation, to ultrasound, a form of nonionizing radiation:

> **Whereas ionizing radiations have well-developed parameters for relating exposure (the amount of ionization produced in air, with units of roentgens) and the dose (the amount of energy deposited per kilogram in the region of interest (units of rads)), medical ultrasound makes no such distinction, with the terms exposure and dose being used (mistakenly) interchangeably.**[25]

The lack of a universal dose quantity is important when attempting to implement ALARA, a safety principle that recommends minimizing exposure. Without a standard measurement of dose, "there is no defined dose which one could systematically lower."[26]

The Inadequacy of the "Safety Controls"

Describing another important deficiency of the "safety controls," Church and Barnett state that the thermal index "does not consider the effect of dwell time, i.e. duration of temperature increase at a single point in tissue."[27] "This is an important failing of the TI because the harm resulting from a temperature elevation depends not only on the magnitude of the elevation but also on the duration of exposure."[28] The risk of tissue damage increases with the duration of exposure, yet the operator has no visual signal that an exposure is excessively long. "One needs to keep in mind that, even with B-mode, dwell time is important as prolonged examination can result in higher exposure levels."[29] Abramowicz writes, "Dwell time is directly under control of the examiner. . . . Since it takes only one pulse to induce cavitation, and about a minute to raise temperature to its peak, time is very important."[30] To minimize risks, he advises, "the best recommendation is to be aware of bioeffects, to perform ultrasound only with a clear medical indication, and to watch TI, MI and the clock."[31]

In a discussion of "the three important parameters under end-user control," Abramowicz identifies a safety lapse that occurs during system setup:

> **Starting or default power is often very high to allow better imaging and end-users will, generally, keep it as such, mostly out of lack of concern for bioeffects.**[32]

It is commonly assumed that prenatal ultrasound is unlikely to produce harmful effects when the power settings are kept low. It is impracticable to do this; the on-screen indices do not provide sufficient information to determine the exact level of exposure. In 2012 the World Federation for Ultrasound in Medicine and Biology recommended that ultrasound scanners used in obstetrics be set to a default power that "should result in a TI no higher than 0.7."[33] This means the thermal index does not predict a fetal temperature rise of more than 0.7 degrees Centigrade. However, as asserted below by many scientists, the thermal and mechanical indices do not present an accurate or complete reading and are difficult to interpret.

According to ultrasound physicists Adam Shaw, of the Acoustics and Ionizing Radiation Division of the National Physical Laboratory (U.K.), and Kevin Martin, Ph.D., FIPEM, "It is tempting but completely wrong to suppose that the on-screen MI and TI is enough to somehow 'characterize' the exposure."[34] The thermal and mechanical indices are "not true safety indices," according to Church and Barnett, because "no particular value is directly related to any quantifiable level of risk of doing harm to the patient."[35] "Because exponential relationships are not intuitive to many users, there is a significant potential for underestimation of the thermal risk associated with exposure to diagnostic ultrasound."[36]

> **It needs to be made very clear that *TI does not represent an actual or an assumed temperature increase.* It bears some correlation with temperature rise in degrees Celsius but in no way allows an estimate or a guess as to what that temperature change *actually* is in the tissue.[37]**
>
> **It has been shown that the TI can underestimate the actual temperature increase in tissue and that manufacturer estimates of intensity, on which the TI is based, can also be significantly in error (Jago et al., 1995).[38]**
>
> **For many of the scanning modes . . . the TI formulations only relate to the risk of thermal damage at the surface near the transducer. If the risk deeper in the tissue were also known, the clinician or sonographer could potentially better assess the**

risk/benefit of increasing the exposure during fetal examinations.[39]

A particular criticism of TI is that it ignores the self-heating of the transducer, and so greatly underestimates the temperature rise within about 5mm of the transducer.[40]

The mechanical index is also considered insufficient because it does not account for all possible mechanical effects, which include "radiation pressure, radiation force, radiation torque, and acoustic streaming"[41]:

[A] simple analysis of another potential mechanism for biological effects, radiation force, indicates that the very form of the MI does not include all non-thermal mechanisms but, perhaps, only one. These results cast doubt on the value of the MI as a reliable means of assessing patient safety.[42]

If Prenatal Ultrasound Is Safe in a Medical Clinic, Why Isn't It Safe in a Commercial Boutique?

Professional associations dedicated to ultrasound safety have issued cautionary statements about nonmedical purveyors of "souvenir," "keepsake," or "bonding" ultrasound images and videos.

The WFUMB disapproves of the use of ultrasound for the sole purpose of providing souvenir images of the fetus. *Because the safety of an ultrasound examination cannot be assured,* the use of ultrasound without medical benefit should be avoided. Furthermore, ultrasound should be employed only

> **by health professionals who are well trained and updated in ultrasound clinical usage and bio-effects.[43] [Emphasis added]**
>
> **—World Federation for Ultrasound in Medicine and Biology (2008)**

> **In the [sic] light of the widespread use of ultrasound in medical practice and its increasing use for "souvenir" fetal imaging commercially, and given the unconfirmed indications from the biological and epidemiological literature of possible neurological effects of in utero ultrasound exposures, there is a need for further research on whether there are any long-term adverse effects of diagnostic ultrasound exposure.[44]**

Although ultrasound equipment is regulated by the FDA's Center for Devices and Radiological Health, "FDA does not regulate how health professionals actually use the equipment."[45] The agency warns:

> **[P]ersons who promote, sell or lease ultrasound equipment for making keepsake fetal videos should know that FDA views this as an unapproved use of a medical device. In addition, those who subject individuals to ultrasound exposure using a diagnostic ultrasound device (a prescription device) without a physician's order may be in violation of State or local laws or regulations regarding use of a prescription medical device.[46]**

In 2009 the State of Connecticut became the first to outlaw the use of entertainment ultrasound. Joshua A. Copel, M.D., professor of obstetrics, gynecology, and reproductive sciences at Yale University and later president of AIUM, wrote a letter in support of Connecticut's introduction of House Bill 5635. It states, in pertinent part:

> **The AIUM and the professional medical community have been concerned about the profusion of storefront entertainment ultrasound facilities for a number of years. Operating in a grey zone at the fringe of medical practice, they raise a number of important issues. While most of us who use clinical ultrasound believe that there is minimal risk in pregnancy when properly calibrated machines are used at appropriate power levels for short periods of time, the machines used at these non-medical facilities are bought from unknown sources and are not required to undergo any specific maintenance or ensure proper performance. The individuals performing the scans may or may not be trained professional sonographers, so there is no way to ascertain their knowledge of the potential for ultrasound bioeffects on the developing fetus, or their ability or willingness to practice safe sonography.**[47]

It should be noted that Copel raises a safety issue that is often neglected: the proper calibration of ultrasound equipment. Shaw and Martin argue that "every medical physics department with an ultrasound responsibility should be capable of validating the displayed indices and should do this as part of acceptance testing when scanners are purchased. Users are expected to make risk-benefit judgements based on the values displayed and need to be reassured that they are reliable."[48] This procedure is "a duty of care to those being scanned" and is necessary "to ensure that equipment is 'fit for purpose,' meets all necessary standards and is properly maintained."[49]

The Rakic Lab's 2006 experiment, described in the previous chapter, explicitly discussed entertainment ultrasound. The researchers assert that in the experiment "the ultrasound parameters and total exposure time are comparable with or below those used by commercial medically nonindicated prenatal ultrasound videos." They conclude, "Therefore our results in pregnant mice support the recommendations by the Food and Drug Administration that warn against the use of medically nonindicated or commercial prenatal ultrasound videos (44)."[50]

Assumptions about the Safety of Ultrasound

> *"Is this safe for my baby?" is a question almost everyone performing obstetric scans has heard. The answer that most will give is, "Of course, it is." This may, in fact, be the correct answer. However, in most cases, this response is more intuitive than based on the examiner's knowledge.*[51]
>
> —Jacques S. Abramowicz, M.D.

Scientific papers often refer to "assumptions" in the field of prenatal ultrasound. For example, it is generally assumed that the benefits of this exam outweigh the risk. Ter Haar evaluates this view:

> **Only if the ratio of risk to benefit is beneficial to the subject can it be considered ethical. The assumption hitherto has always been that ultrasound scans are "safe". There are a number of reasons not to be blasé about ultrasound safety. Firstly, it is well known that ultrasound can be used to produce changes in biological tissue—it is this that drives its use as a therapeutic agent, whether at low powers for physiotherapy or drug delivery, or at higher powers for cancer therapy where instantaneous cell killing is sought. Can we really be sure that the ultrasound**

pulsing regimes used in ultrasound imaging are not also producing biological changes that may be considered deleterious in the context of an imaging application?

Secondly . . . while existing human epidemiological studies of the safety of ultrasound are reassuring, it must be remembered that the scans under consideration for these [studies] were all carried out using early clinical scanners, before the increase in output levels that has taken place over the last two decades.[52]

In a consensus report, the Bioeffects Committee of the American Institute of Ultrasound in Medicine reveals an important consequence of the medical profession's assumption of safety: "The assumption of safety regulated ultrasound may have contributed to the general lack of adoption of the ALARA (as low as reasonably achievable) principle to obtain the necessary diagnostic information and the use of the TI and mechanical index (MI) as feedback to the operator on safety."[53] The first line of ter Haar's preface to *The Safe Use of Ultrasound in Medical Diagnosis* reads, "It is an oft-observed fact that safety sessions at congresses are seldom well attended . . . but the fact remains that the safe use of diagnostic ultrasound is the responsibility of the person conducting the scan."[54]

Abramowicz paraphrases the attitude of physicians who feel it is unnecessary to further their knowledge of ultrasound safety: "'It is a well-known fact that ultrasound is safe and I use an [sic] Food and Drug Administration (FDA)-approved instrument so I have nothing to fear and reading this chapter or similar chapters in other books is a waste of time.'" He counters:

Regarding the fact that the machines are "FDA approved," although it is correct that the US FDA has

imposed limits to the acoustic outputs of ultrasound instruments, the power emitted by the machine is under direct control of the examiner and, based on the application chosen (such as spectral Doppler) and control changes (eg, focal length or gate size), this output can vary greatly, to levels potentially known to have detrimental consequences.[55]

The fetus may be exposed to hazardous levels of ultrasound in the hospital or the doctor's office, as well as in storefront businesses. It is well known that ultrasound can cause a rise in temperature in fetal tissue. In an example of excessive use, Abramowicz, Barnett, Duck, *et al.*, state:

Whenever a pregnant woman visits her obstetrician, and the woman is febrile, the obstetrician will often scan the fetus just to be sure that "everything is OK," thereby increasing the thermal load to the fetus.[56]

According to Abramowicz, the assumption of safety is often based on the belief that ultrasound, in contrast to x-ray, poses no risk of harm to human tissue:

If asked, the vast majority of end users (and patients) will respond that ultrasound is not X-rays and is completely safe. In reality, there is a marked lack of knowledge on effects of ultrasound in tissues being examined (bioeffects) among the majority of these end-users.(5)[57]

In 2001 O'Brien and Siddiqi expressed scientists' ongoing concern that frequent exposure to ultrasound, and increased dose and duration of exposure, produce subtle adverse effects in humans:

> **Based on the fact that results of experimental studies have proven inconsistent, it is clear that the interaction of ultrasound with biological systems, in particular those with rapidly dividing cells, is still not fully understood.** ***What remains of concern are the subtle and long-term manifestations of frequent intrauterine exposure.*** **These concerns remain pertinent due to a number of factors such as the continued rise in the percentage of the prenatal population that is exposed each year and advances in technology that can result in increased exposure (dose) to the fetus. The exposure time may also be increased as additional diagnostic information is sought. These points emphasize the need to pursue these questions in an effort to confirm that unwanted effects do not occur.[58]**

Duck summarizes the reasons why no scientist can vouch for the safety of prenatal ultrasound with confidence:

> **There are deficiencies in the safety indices as appropriate and only means to monitor safety. The physical models are simplistic; the predictive ability for a temperature rise is questionable; and the user is given no information about transducer self-heating. In addition, knowledge about the safety implications of ultrasound exposure is still limited. Thermal teratologic studies are still being reinterpreted; recent epidemiologic evidence on handedness is still under review; and there is almost no knowledge of the direct effects of radiation stress on cell behavior. It would be unethical to transfer responsibility for safety to the user on the basis of such incomplete and potentially misleading information.[59]**

Ultrasound scientists agree that the safety of prenatal ultrasound cannot be assured. While expectant mothers find reassurance in a standard safety statement, the disquieting concerns of the scientific community will not be silenced. Ultrasound experts warn that prenatal ultrasound may cause subtle or delayed effects. A small aberration in the developing brain can produce the behavioral symptoms characteristic of ASD. The damage is demonstrated by the behavior of the child only as time passes. Ultrasound is capable of causing the brain to develop along a different path than that ordained by nature.

Under today's clinical conditions, prenatal ultrasound is never performed without risk to the fetal brain. The developing brain is especially vulnerable to heating, the primary effect of ultrasound. The skull bone heats rapidly, and it does not take long to produce irreversible damage to the cerebral cortex beneath. Since 1976, unborn children have been subjected to increasing intensities of ultrasound. It is well known that safety measures have not kept pace with this "hot" technology.[60] To date, we have no standard measurement of a dose of ultrasound radiation. We are unable to calculate precisely how long a region of fetal tissue has been exposed. The "so-called 'safety indices'"[61], intended to warn the operator of excessive exposure, do not permit an estimate of the temperature rise in fetal tissue. The operator, who is solely responsible for the safety of the sonogram, lacks both the tools and the knowledge to implement the principle of ALARA. Despite the "gaps in our knowledge about ultrasound safety,"[62] prenatal ultrasound is used under a false assumption of safety and virtually without regulation worldwide.

Autism spectrum disorder is often depicted as a puzzle[63]—a disease without a known cause or cure. Its cause is no longer a mystery when we realize our unborn children are repeatedly exposed to hazardous levels of ultrasound without adequate safeguards. The terms *autism* and *ASD* mask the true nature of the epidemic. We are witnessing traumatic brain injury inflicted by ultrasound. In the history of medicine, many accepted practices have been abandoned when they proved harmful. We cannot entrust the well being of future generations to ultrasound, with its known risks. The upward trend of ultrasound and autism can be reversed by following the adage at the head of this chapter:

> ***The use of ultrasound without a medical indication to view the fetus, obtain images of the fetus or determine the fetal gender is inappropriate and contrary to responsible medical practice.***[64]
>
> **—American Institute of Ultrasound in Medicine, 2012**

ENDNOTES
III. The "Uncharted Waters" of Ultrasound Safety

1. American Institute for Ultrasound in Medicine. AIUM Official Statement: Prudent Use in Pregnancy (2012), cited in Abramowicz, J. S. (2012), Bioeffects of obstetric ultrasound for the clinician: How to keep it safe. Institute for Advanced Medical Education, p. 11. Retrieved on 22 July 2013 from https://iame.com/online/bioeffects_of_obstetric_ultrasound/content.php.

2. American Institute of Ultrasound in Medicine (2013). AIUM Practice Guideline for the Performance of Obstetric Ultrasound Examinations. Retrieved from http://www.aium.org/resources/guidelines/obstetric.pdf. Indications for first trimester are listed on p. 3; indications for second and third trimesters, on p. 6.

3. Ter Haar, G. [Ed.] (2012). Introduction, *The Safe Use of Ultrasound in Medical Diagnosis,* p. 1. Retrieved from http://www.birjournals.org/site/book/Safe_Use_of_Ultrasound.pdf.

4. Ter Haar, G. [Ed.] (2012). Preface, *The Safe Use of Ultrasound in Medical Diagnosis,* p. v.

5. AIUM Safety Statement (approved 27 March 2010). "Conclusions Regarding Epidemiology for Obstetric Ultrasound." Retrieved 2 September 2014 from http://www.aium.org/ On home page, click on Official Statements to view this and other safety statements regarding ultrasound in pregnancy.

6. The Mayo Clinic. Fetal ultrasound. This 2012 document was still on the Internet in December 2014. Retrieved from http://www.mayoclinic.org/tests-procedures/fetal-ultrasound/basics/risks/prc-20014506.

7. Kaiser Permanente—Regional Health Education—"Ultrasound Exam in Pregnancy" E-Handout #7326-E (Revised 7-08) RL 102. This 2008 document was still on the Internet in December 2014. Originally retrieved but no longer accessible at http://mydoctor.kaiserpermanente.org/ncal/Images/GEN_Ultrasound_Exam_in_Pregnancy_10-10_tcm63-9059.pdf. The description of risk has been revised since 2008. In "Prenatal Services," a Kaiser Permanente publication last reviewed in January

2013, the following language appears under Risks: "Ultrasound has been routinely used in pregnancy since the 1960s. Based on a large number of medical studies, there are no known health risks to the fetus or mother associated with routine use of prenatal ultrasound." Retrieved from http://mydoctor.kaiserpermanente.org/ncal/specialty/genetics/prenatal_services/ In Prenatal Services box on right, click on Prenatal Ultrasound; see Risks.

8. Tarantal, A. F., O'Brien, W. D. Jr., Hendrickx, A. G. (1993). Evaluation of the bioeffects of prenatal ultrasound exposure in the cynomolgus macaque (macaca fascicularis): III. Developmental and hematologic studies. *Teratology,* vol. 47, p. 159.

9. Abramowicz, J. S. (2013). Bioeffects of obstetric ultrasound for the clinician: How to keep it safe, p. 1. Institute for Advanced Medical Education. Retrieved from https://iame.com/online/bioeffects_of_obstetric_ultrasound/content.php.

10. Ibid., p. 15.

11. Abramowicz, J. S. (2007). Editorial: Prenatal exposure to ltrasound waves: Is there a risk? *Ultrasound in Obstetrics and Gynecology,* vol. 29, p. 366.

12. Duck, F. A. (1999). Is it safe to use diagnostic ultrasound during the first trimester? *Ultrasound in Obstetrics and Gynecology*, vol. 13, p. 385.

13. Abramowicz, J. S., Lewin, P. A., and Goldberg, B. (2011). Ultrasound bioeffects for the perinatologist, p. 8. Global Library of Women's Medicine (ISSN: 1756-2228) 2011. doi:10.3843/GLOWM.10204. The exact quote is as follows: "With the higher limits comes the potential for increased risk to the patient, so the clinician must make a careful risk/benefit analysis."

14. O'Brien, W. D. (1998). Assessing the risks for modern diagnostic ultrasound imaging, p. 20. Retrieved from http://www.brl/uiuc.edu/Projects/Bioeffects/Asessing,php.

15. Sheiner, E., Shoham-Vardi, I., and Abramowicz, J. S. (2007). What do clinical users know regarding safety of ultrasound during pregnancy? *Journal of Ultrasound in Medicine,* vol. 26, p. 2. Retrieved from http://www.jultrasoundmed.org/content/26/3/319.

16. Ter Haar writes: "The passage of an ultrasonic pressure wave

through tissue also leads to 'mechanical' effects. These include acoustic cavitation and phenomena arising from radiation pressure effects, such as acoustic streaming. It is acoustic streaming that is of most concern on safety grounds." This statement is followed by a definition of cavitation. Ter Haar, G. (2011). Ultrasonic imaging: Safety considerations, p. 688. Interface Focus. Retrieved from http://rsfs.royalsocietypublishing.org/content/1/4/686.full.htlm#related-urls. doi:10.1098/rsfs.2011.0029.

17. Duck, F. A. (1999). Ultrasound exposure measurement: A hidden science? *The British Journal of Radiology,* vol. 78, p. 290.

18. Abramowicz, J. S. (2014). Ultrasound in reproductive medicine: Is it safe? in Stadtmauer, L. A., and Tur-Kaspa, I. [Eds.], *Ultrasound Imaging in Reproductive Medicine* (New York: Springer Science + Business Media], p. 7. doi: 10.1007/978-1-4614-9182-8_1.

19. O'Brien, W. D. (1998). Assessing the risks of diagnostic ultrasound imaging, p. 21. Retrieved from http://www.brl/uiuc.edu/Projects/Bioeffects/Asessing,php.

20. Caviness, S., and Grant, P. E. (2006). Our unborn children at risk? Proceedings of the National Academy of Sciences, v. 103, pp. 12661-62. Retrieved from http://www.pnas.org/content/103/34/12661.full. (p. 3)

21. U.S. Food and Drug Administration (2013). ALARA Education Program. Guidance for Industry and FDA Staff – Information for Manufacturers Seeking Marketing Clearance of Diagnostic Ultrasound Systems and Transducers, pp. 35-36. Retrieved from http://www.fda.gov/medicaldevices/deviceregulationandguidance/guidancedocuments/ucm089001.

22. Abramowicz, J. S. (2010). Fetal Doppler: How to keep it safe? *Clinical Obstetrics and Gynecology*, vol. 53, p. 845.

23. Maršál, K. (2005). The output display: Has it missed its target? *Ultrasound in Obstetrics and Gynecology*, vol. 25, p. 213.

24. Duck, F. A. (2005). Ultrasound exposure measurement: A hidden science? *The British Journal of Radiology,* vol. 78, p. 289.

25. Ter Haar, G. (2011). Ultrasonic imaging: Safety considerations, p. 689. *Interface Focus 2011 1,* doi:10.1098/rsfs/2011.0029.

26. Miller, D. L. (2008). Safety assurance in obstetric ultrasound. *Seminars in Ultrasound, CT, and MRI,* 29(2), p. 10.

27. Church, C. C., and Barnett, S. B. (2012). Ultrasound-induced heating and its biological consequences, in *The Safe Use of Ultrasound in Medical Diagnosis,* p. 48. Retrieved from http://www.birjournals.org/site/book/Safe_Use_of_Ultrasound.pdf. Church and Barnett explain on page 62 of their paper, "The TI [Thermal Index] does not include time as one of its input parameters. This simplification is necessary owing to the severe technical challenges that must be met and the enormous computational overhead required for a diagnostic machine to determine exactly when it began imaging a region of tissue and when it has been moved to a different region. Various possible solutions to the problem have been proposed (Lubbers et al., 2003; Church, 2007; Ziskin, 2010), but none has yet been adopted by any regulatory agency or manufacturer."

28. Ziskin, M. C. (2010). The thermal dose index. *Journal of Ultrasound in Medicine,* vol. 29, p. 1476. Ziskin proposes a solution in this paper.

29. Abramowicz, J. S. (2010). Fetal Doppler: How to keep it safe. *Clinical Obstetrics and Gynecology,* vol. 53, no. 4, p. 848.

30. Abramowicz, J. S. (2008). Bioeffects of obstetric ultrasound for the clinician: How to keep it safe, p. 3. Institute for Advanced Medical Education, retrieved from https://iame.com/online/bioeffects of obstetric ultrasound/content.php.

31. Ibid., p. 9.

32. Abramowicz, J. S. (2008). Bioeffects of obstetric ultrasound for the clinician: How to keep it safe, p. 3. Institute for Advanced Medical Education, retrieved from https://iame.com/online/bioeffects of obstetric ultrasound/content.php.

33. World Federation for Ultrasound in Medicine and Biology (2012), WFUMB Clinical Safety Statement for Diagnostic Ultrasound—An Overview. Retrieved from http://www.wfumb.org/about/statements.aspx. Under Safety Statements, click on title.

34. Shaw, A., and Martin, K. (2012). The acoustic output of diagnostic ultrasound scanners, in *The Safe Use of Ultrasound in Medical Diagnosis,* p. 24.

35. Church, C. C., and Barnett, S. (2012). Ultrasound-induced heating and its biological consequences, in *The Safe Use of Ultrasound in*

Medical Diagnosis, pp. 61-62.

36. Church, C. C. (2007). A proposal to clarify the relationship between the thermal index and the corresponding risk to the patient, *Ultrasound in Medicine and Biology*, p. 1489. Retrieved from http://www.umbjournal.org/article/S0301-5629(07)00134-2/abstract.

37. Abramowicz, J. S., Lewin, P. A., and Goldberg, B. B. (2011). Ultrasound bioeffects for the perinatologist, p. 9. Global Library of Women's Medicine, (ISSN: 1756-2228) 2011. doi: 10.3843/GLOWM.10204.

38. Church, C. C., and Barnett, S. B. (2012). Ultrasound-induced heating and its biological consequences, in *The Safe Use of Ultrasound in Medical Diagnosis*, p. 48. Retrieved from http://www.birjournals.org/site/book/Safe_Use_of_Ultrasound.pdf.

39. Bigelow, T. A., Church, C. C., Sandstrom, K., Abbott, J. G., Ziskin, M.C., et al. (2011). The thermal index: Its strengths, weaknesses, and proposed improvements. *Journal of Ultrasound in Medicine*, vol. 30, no. 5, p. 714. Retrieved from http://www.jultrasoundmed.org/content/30/5/714.long. (See p. 8)

40. Shaw, A., and Martin, K. (2012). The acoustic output of diagnostic ultrasound scanners, in *The Safe Use of Ultrasound in Medical Diagnosis*, p. 22.

41. Lewin, P. A., and Goldberg, B. B. (2011). Ultrasound bioeffects for the perinatologist, chapter 71, p. 3. Retrieved from http://www.glowm.com/resources/glowm/cd/pages/v3/v3c071.html.

42. Church, C. C. (2013). The mechanical index and bubbles in tissue, an evidentiary review. *Journal of the Acoustic Society of America*, Nov. 2013; 134(5):3975. doi:10.1121/1.4830482.

43. WFUMB Policy Statement on Non-medical Use of Ultrasound (2008), in *The Safe Use of Ultrasound in Medical Diagnosis*, p. 155.

44. Report of the Independent Advisory Group on Non-ionising Radiation, Documents of the Health Protection Agency (2010), *Health Effects of Exposure to Ultrasound and Infrasound*, p. 4. Retrieved from http://www.hpa.org.uk/webc/HPAWebFile/HPAweb_C/1265028759369.

45. FDA Consumer Health Information (2008). Taking a close look at ultrasound. Retrieved from http://www.fda.gov/downloads/

ForConsumers/consumerupdates/UCM095487.pdf.

46. U.S. Food and Drug Administration (2005). Patient Alerts: Fetal Keepsake Videos. Retrieved from http://www.fda/gov/MedicalDevices/Safety/Alertsandnotices/PatientAlerts/ Click on Fetal Keepsake Videos.

47. Copel, J. A. (2009). Letter to Connecticut representatives Pat Widlitz and Deborah Heinrich. Retrieved from http://www.cga.ct.gov/2009/PHdata/Tmy/2009HB-05635-R000227-joshua.

48. Shaw, A., and Martin, K. (2012). The acoustic output of diagnostic ultrasound scanners, in *The Safe Use of Ultrasound in Medical Diagnosis,* p. 41.

49. Ibid., p. 24.

50. Ang, ESBC Jr., Cluncic, V., Duque, A., Schafer, M.E., and Rakic, P. Prenatal exposure to ultrasound waves impacts neuronal migration in mice, p. 12908. Retrieved from http://www.pnas.org/cgi/doi/10.1073/pnas.0605294103.

51. Abramowicz, J. S. (2002). Ultrasound in obstetrics and gynecology: Is this hot technology too hot? *Journal of Ultrasound in Medicine,* vol. 21, no. 12, p. 1327.

52. Ter Haar, G. (Ed.) (2011). Ultrasonic imaging: Safety considerations, p. 686. Interface Focus. Retrieved from http://rsfs.royalsocietypublishing.org/content/1/4/686.full.html#related-urls.

53. Bioeffects Committee of the American Institute of Ultrasound in Medicine (2008). American Institute of Ultrasound in Medicine Consensus Report on Potential Bioeffects of Diagnostic Ultrasound: Executive Summary. *Journal of Ultrasound in Medicine,* vol. 27, April 2008, pp. 504-505. Retrieved from http://www.jultrasoundmed.org/content/27/4/503.full.pdf.

54. Ter Haar, G. [Ed.] (2012). Preface, *The Safe Use of Ultrasound in Medicine,* p. v.

55. Abramowicz, J. S. (2010). Fetal Doppler: How to keep it safe? *Clinical Obstetrics and Gynecology,* vol. 53, no. 4, p. 843.

56. Abramowicz, J. S., Barnett, S. B., Duck, F. A., Edmonds, P. D., Hynynen, K. H., Ziskin, M. C. (2008). Fetal thermal effects of diagnostic ultrasound. *Journal of Ultrasound in Medicine*, vol. 27, p. 554.

57. Abramowicz, J. S. Bioeffects of obstetric ultrasound for the

clinician: How to keep it safe (2008), p. 1. Institute for Advanced Medical Education. Retrieved from https://iame.com/online/bioeffects_of_obstetric_ultrasound/content.php.

58. O'Brien, W. D. Jr., and Siddiqi, T. A. Obstetric sonography: The Output Display Standard and ultrasound bioeffects, in *Sonography in Obstetrics and Gynecology: Principles and Practice* (New York: McGraw-Hill, 2001), p. 43.

59. Duck, F. A. (2002), in Acoustic output upper limits proposition: Should upper limits be retained? by O'Brien, W. D., Abbott, J. G., Stratmeyer, M. E., Harris, G. R., Schafer, M. E., Siddiqi, T. A., Merritt, C. R. B., Duck, F. A., and Bendick, P. J. *Journal of Ultrasound in Medicine,* vol. 21, p. 1340.

60. This refers to the title of Abramowicz's 2002 paper Is this hot technology too hot? *Journal of Ultrasound in Medicine,* vol. 21, no. 12, pp. 1327-1333.

61. Duck, F. A. (1999). Ultrasound exposure measurement: A hidden science? *The British Journal of Radiology,* vol. 78, p. 290.

62. Ter Haar, G. [Ed.] (2012). Preface, *The Safe Use of Ultrasound in Medical Diagnosis,* p. v.

63. "The Autism Awareness Puzzle," a puzzle twisted into a ribbon, "is the most recognized symbol of the autism community," according to the Autism Society of America. See http://www.autism-society.org/get-involved/national-autism-awareness-month/

64. American Institute for Ultrasound in Medicine. AIUM Official Statement: Prudent Use in Pregnancy (2012), cited in Abramowicz, J. S. (2012), Bioeffects of obstetric ultrasound for the clinician: How to keep it safe? Institute for Advanced Medical Education, p. 11. Retrieved from https://iame.com/online/bioeffects_of_obstetric_ultrasound/content.php.